MISGUIDED MEDICINE

MISGUIDED MEDICINE

Colin E. Champ, M.D.

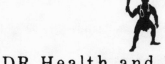

CDR Health and Nutrition, LLC
Pittsburgh

Copyright © 2014 CDR Health and Nutrition, LLC

Published by CDR Health and Nutrition, LLC
Editing by Megan Mischler
Cover design by Scott Nicklos
Author photographs by Dan Landoni
Book design and formatting by Megan Mischler

The material contained within this book is strictly for
informational and educational purposes only and is not
intended or implied to be a substitute for professional
medical advice, diagnosis, or treatment. If you have questions
about your medical condition, you should seek the advice of
a physician or qualified health provider. We urge you to not
disregard, avoid, or delay in obtaining professional medical
advice because of something you have read in this book. All
usage of the information presented here is at the reader's
discretion and the author specifically disclaims any and all
liability arising directly or indirectly from the usage of any
and all information contained within.

All rights reserved. No part of this book may be reproduced,
stored in a retrieval system, transmitted in any form or by
any means, mechanical or electronic, including recording,
photocopying, scanning, or by any storage system without
written permission by the author.

Printed by CreateSpace, An Amazon.com Company
Manufactured in the United States of America

For information about special discounts for bulk purchases
or to book an event with the author contact
Megan Mischler at megan@cavemandoctor.com

ISBN 13: 978-1500675387
ISBN 10: 1500675385

To

JOHN REICHL (1917-2014),
*who taught me at a young age and throughout my life
about the importance of taking my wellbeing into my own hands
by staying healthy both physically and mentally.*

CONTENTS

PREFACE

During my studies at the Massachusetts Institute of Technology, I was taught to think. Our tests were open book and anything that could be found in a reference book was never asked of us. My intense and valuable medical training was drastically different, as it required the memorization of immense amounts of information. While appropriate, this often led to me blindly following what was taught to me without question. Part of this training taught my colleagues to avoid asking questions and focus on regurgitating the information instead.

Sometimes physicians, patients, and even scientists forget to ask questions and challenge what they are taught or what they may already know. Such events lead to the perpetuation of information that is often incorrect. This book was compiled during my constant assessment of what I was being taught, and what I was supposed to pass on to patients as healthy recommendations.

As I took an oath to "prescribe regimens for the good of my patients according to my ability and my judgment and never do harm to anyone," I took such learning very seriously, and in doing so decided to write this book to ensure that others abide by this rule as well. I also realized the importance of each and every one of my patients taking an active role in their health and being their own physician first, then calling for help when needed.

Colin E. Champ, M.D.

ACKNOWLEDGMENTS

I would like to thank all those who were instrumental in the creation and inspiration of this book. Growing up in a large Italian family, the importance of food was prevalent from day one, and for that I would thank Regis, Cynthia, Christian, and Chelsey Champ; John and Rose (Pesce) Reichl; Mary Ann, Mark, Debbie, Frank, and Erica Zappala; Cloe and Joe Cirilano; and Justin, Julia, Mary and Les Broglie for imparting the important social, cultural, and health aspects of food. Megan Mischler was invaluable in the editing and design of the book as well as making the science less sciency.

I would also like to thank all those who were instrumental in my learning and motivation regarding the importance of diet and exercise in health care, including Dr. Mark Mishra, Roger Dickerman, Dr. Gene Fine, Dr. Rainer Klement, Dr. Jeff Volek, Dr. Timothy Showalter, Dr. Sebastian Heersink, Dr. Joshua Siglin, Dr. Steve Stache, Dr. Nitin Ohri, Dr. Tu Dan, Dr. Joshua Palmer, Dr. Nicole Simone, Dr. Maria Werner-Wasik, Dr. Pramila Rani Anné, Keith and Michele Norris, Dr. Renato Baserga, and Dr. Tommy Haytmanek.

MISGUIDED MEDICINE

"One of the first duties of the physician is to educate the masses not to take medicine."

—*William Osler,*
Founding Father of
Johns Hopkins Hospital

INTRODUCTION

Fifty percent of medicine is wrong.[1] You read that right; however, we have known for years that medicine is part science
and part art, and any model with as many variables as the
human body is nearly impossible to master. This is not necessarily the fault of the treating physician, or even medicine
itself, but rather a combination of the scientific method, bias,
financial incentive, and of course, the human drive to advance science. In fact, many, if not most, medical studies are
doomed to fail from the start,[2] with the final result leaving
most physicians more confused than before the study even
took place. When the press gets wind of these studies, this
confusion is only amplified at an alarming pace.

In actuality, *wrong* may be a strong word. More appropriately, medicine is often *unfounded*. In other words, medical findings are often premature and need refining. Unfortunately, in our mass media and mass-produced society,
these undeveloped findings often become "science" before
they were ever analyzed and polished. Much like opening a
fine wine before it has matured; these results are exposed too
soon; yet end up in doctors' offices as recommendations, or
worse yet, by insurance companies as mandates for coverage.

This leads to changing recommendations on nearly a daily basis. One day fiber is extremely beneficial for one's health;
the next day it is irrelevant. In fact, over fifty percent of even
high-level studies will actually contradict themselves at some
point in the future.[3]

As a physician, such information is tenuous. Basically,
when a doctor recommends a treatment to a patient based
on a randomized trial, he or she will theoretically be providing them with incorrect recommendations nearly every other

time. Flip a coin and the patient may derive the same benefit.

Whether choosing to avoid flipping a coin to decide one's health or simply deciding to assume a proactive approach, it becomes clear that the pathway to health must be taken in the patient's own hands. While physicians clearly provide benefit to aid in preventative care along with support once pathology occurs, real health is derived from proactively taking health into one's own hands, not under the control of others who, unknowingly, may be flipping a coin to decide what is best. Others may be able to guide individuals, but real health lies within.

The easy way to avoid the vulnerable areas of science and medicine that are ever-changing on a daily basis is to ignore them. More specifically, watching such changes with a bird's-eye view while the science "ripens" and mimicking the lifestyle habits of those that have worked for centuries may be the safest bet. However, to follow such a lifestyle would rely on one taking his or her health into his or her own hands by staying informed of the latest scientific findings while continuing in a "common-sense" fashion to follow the aspects that have worked for centuries to keep individuals free of modern diseases, like obesity, diabetes, heart disease, and cancer.

Much like the government and other institutions, once a policy is established, it is near impossible to remove or even change. During medical school, which was not too long ago for me, I spent over $300,000 to learn science, medicine, and unfortunately, policy backed by little evidence but more often tradition – traditions that, much like unchangeable government policy, get perpetuated for decades with little evidence backing them. Once these traditions gain momentum, it is difficult to stop them. This book refuses to perpetuate these false traditions, and instead, aims to point out the inaccuracies of such falsehoods by analyzing the existing data. In many cases, the data tells us to not only ignore these traditions but often to do the exact opposite.

Medicine

"Medicine is the art of entertaining the patient as the body heals itself."

–Voltaire

Medicine is the youngest science of all. Medicine must continually balance attempts to evaluate scientific hypotheses, while allowing these hypotheses to become truths. Such a balance is challenging to manage and often faulty hypotheses become faulty truths. This occurs in good nature, as patients continually push for new treatments and physicians continually push to advance the fight against disease. Medicine is a great science that is helping humanity progress and increasing our lifespan at a rapid rate.

Accordingly, reverence for the institute of medicine has persisted throughout the years. Doctors navigate the sterile hallways of the white-walled hospitals in their white coats, resembling that of scientists. However, we must remember that medicine is not only science, but rather part science and part art. Or better yet, a majority is art with a touch of science.

This book is not putting the blame of these mistakes on doctors, as they clearly do not know all the answers and are required to make decisions based on the available data. However, often times the available data are merely recommendations contrived from government committees or pushed by the industry that is set out to receive large financial rewards and backed by little credible science. While mistakes are common in an imperfect science and must be forgiven, several are too blatantly wrong to ignore and are leading to the downfall of many aspects of our health. Yet, these are likely recommendations that you have heard incessantly over the past several decades or even your lifetime. Unfortunately, many of these recommendations and wrong advice continue to get perpetuated by the medical field, continually promoting unhealthy lifestyle habits.

This book explores these recommendations, debunks them, and provides you with actual tangible methods to achieve optimal health, or at least allows you to make your own conclusions as to which methods promote health and which restrict it. This work aims to provide the reader with the knowhow to avoid the daily back and forth of the media regarding scientific findings, and instead, take one's health into his or her own hands.

The goal of this book is to take you along the journey of how and why we got it wrong in several main areas of health. In doing so, the data as to how and why we got it wrong is provided including all necessary references. Providing the data is a necessity, but due to its tediousness, it has been limited only to the necessary amount. If you would like to research any area further, simply follow the reference in the bibliography section.

PART ONE

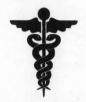

THE FORMATION OF THE STANDARD AMERICAN DIET

High Carbohydrates, Endorsing Grains, Counting Calories, and Chastising Fat

---

"The diet-heart idea – the notion that saturated fats and cholesterol cause heart disease – is the greatest scientific deception of our times."
  –Dr. George Mann,
    co-director Framingham Health Study

THE WAR ON FAT

*F*or several decades, it was thought that simply consuming fewer calories was the clearest path to weight loss and improvements in health. It was also thought that dietary fat was directly converted to fat within the body, and that process is what slows blood flow through the arteries and accumulates within them, leading to cardiovascular disease and heart attacks. As a result, the war on dietary fat was waged.

Conceptually, this was an easy target as a logical explanation of fat accumulation in the body was the result of fat consumed in the diet. Unfortunately, this was not the case physiologically, and as is often the case, without physiologic support, there was no scientific support to back up such claims that fat was making us fat, clogging our arteries, or leading the U.S. population along the pathway to metabolic derangement. In fact, the increase in obesity and metabolic disorders has followed a reduction of fat within the diet over the past three decades.[4-6] Yet, the placement of the crosshairs on fat as enemy number one was rather easy.

This story begins in the early 1900s with the Russian scientist, Nikolai Anichkov, and a rabbit. In a series of experiments, Anichkov found that rabbits developed atherosclerosis, or clogged arteries, when their standard vegetable diet was replaced with heavy amounts of cholesterol in the form of meat and eggs.[7] This was the first study to reveal the potential of a high-fat or high-cholesterol diet to result in the accumulation of cholesterol within the arteries. Such findings were clearly groundbreaking.

However, one major roadblock stood in the way of translating this experiment to humans; it was performed in rabbits. As anyone who has watched Sunday cartoons knows, rabbits are vegetarians with little to no fat in their diet.[8-10] Correspondingly, they are nearly incapable of processing heavy fat, as their livers, much *unlike* human livers, are inept at processing excessive quantities of cholesterol. To further complicate this issue, the large intestine of the rabbit dominates in proportion to the stomach, comprising up to forty percent of the digestive tract. Within the large intestine, digestible elements of the diet are separated from the fibrous and the undigested parts, as vegetables often contain many indigestible components. Rabbits then digest food elements within their hindgut.

All of these physiologic and anatomic differences between the rabbit and human largely questioned these data from the start, if not making it totally irrelevant with regard to humans. Nevertheless, later studies confirmed similar results by supplying rabbits with a diet heavy in fat, not just cholesterol, which led to similar accumulation of cholesterol within their arteries.[11] Such studies placed the blame directly on cholesterol and now fat in the diet as the cause of clogged arteries.

Decades later, further experiments were performed with rabbits that were overfed a fatty diet. However, in these studies, a different picture was painted. These studies revealed that cholesterol only accumulated within the arteries that were damaged,[12] sparing healthy arteries. It was also found that mice with clogged arteries had the same cholesterol as those with unclogged arteries, and the only difference between the two groups was that the mice that had foreign material injected into their arteries experienced cholesterol accumulation within these vessels.

These findings questioned whether fat or cholesterol was in fact clogging the arteries or merely coating the damaged areas of the arteries much like a bandage. This begs the question whether the initial accusations were in fact blaming the bandage and ignoring the *cause* of the damage. Further adding to the confusion is the fact that clots within arteries are generally a combination of several materials, including cholesterol, immune cells, and a large amount of calcium; this is why they are seen on medical x-rays and CT scans as calcified plaques.

This arterial damage can occur via several mechanisms, including trauma, inflammation, smoking, stress, and infection. Other data reveals that a specific type of cholesterol, known as oxidized cholesterol, is the culprit of arterial damage.[13] Oxidized cholesterol is cholesterol that contains free radicals. As the body encounters free radicals, they cause havoc resulting in organ damage and even cancer.

One of the many functions of cholesterol is that it appears to bind these elements to offset their potential damage and, as a result, accumulates in areas of damage, once again pointing to cholesterol as the bandage and not the damage itself. Along these lines, individuals with elevated cholesterol may simply be producing more in order to combat an inflammatory state within their body. Interestingly, when rabbits are fed a diet high in cholesterol but also given free radical fighting antioxidants, the arterial damage and clogged arteries are prevented.[14] This data further points to inflammatory damage to arterial walls via free radical damage or oxidation in this case as the culprit and cholesterol as the quick fix.[15]

Clearly avoiding this damage, and not necessarily cholesterol, will be a more efficacious strategy to keep the arteries free of blockages.

These studies also ignore the physiologic importance of cholesterol. In fact, the demonization of fat and cholesterol likely leaves most Americans unsure if there is any benefit to cholesterol; however, without cholesterol, life is impossible. Cholesterol helps form several vital hormones, like vitamin D, which leads to bone strength, a healthy immune system, and the ability to fight cancer. It is not surprising that low cholesterol has been associated with increased cancer risk[16] and increased risk of death.[17]

Champion of Low Fat

Several decades later, Ancel Keys entered the picture. He was a researcher in physiology at the University of Minnesota. His work initially dealt with methods of providing soldiers with high-calorie nonperishable food sources during World War II. The final product of this work was "K-rations" for the military. Furthermore, throughout this work, he became more interested in the body's response to diet, and eventually ran the infamous Minnesota Starvation study, where conscious objectors were studied closely as they underwent a period of starvation.[18]

He agreed that fat was an enemy to health and set out to relay the message to the world.[19,20] Interestingly, supposedly even Keys felt that Anichkov's experiments proved nothing, as he believed that *cholesterol* triggered an inflammatory reaction in the arteries of the rabbits instead of merely accumulating within them.

After the mid-20th century, Keys then performed what is arguably the most controversial study of our time, where he analyzed the fat intake and death rates of humans throughout several countries in the world. While the controversies vary depending on the source, many have accused Keys of cherry-picking his data to support his hypothesis. In his Seven Countries Study, he reported on death rates from heart disease in countries, including Japan, Italy, England, Wales, Australia, Canada, and the United States.[21] Keys found that in these seven countries the more fat that was consumed, the higher the rate of heart disease and death.

To the blind eye, such findings supported Anichkov's initial experiments. However, the details become vague and controversial as Keys apparently had the data available on 22 countries at his disposal, and he conveniently left the data out from other countries that did not support his hypothesis as strongly. Removing these countries apparently strengthened his results, which if true, is clearly unethical and deceiving. Upon assessing fat consumption and cardiovascular death in all 22 countries, the association between fat and heart disease became much smaller and suggested a potential relationship, although no conclusions were made.

Interestingly, the association between protein and heart disease was actually greater, but as he set out to demonize fat, this association was apparently never mentioned publicly. Unfortunately, as this has become such a heated topic between vegan, vegetarian, and other diet groups, it has become difficult to get to the bottom of the real story. Regardless, Keys actually received much criticism in his day for both his findings and his scientific methods. His scientific deception was aptly described by two prominent scientists of the time, Yerushalmey and Hilleboe.[22] They correctly pointed out that many aspects in the diet of *all* the available countries should be assessed, as cherry picking certain elements may be misleading. An even closer look at the data actually reveals that high-fat intake was likely a surrogate marker for industrialization of these countries, which often accompanies an array of health problems in itself.

However, with further assessment of the data, it was

found that higher animal fat and protein consumption were correlated with an increased risk of death from cardiovascular disease. Yet, their consumption actually decreased the risk of both non heart-related and *overall* risk of death. As a result, a high-fat diet may increase the risk of death from heart attack, but would decrease the risk of *overall* death. Upon closer review, the greatest risk of death came in those individuals with the highest consumption of carbohydrates. However, while no definite conclusions can be made from this data as it merely reveals associations, there was little to no mention of the relationship between dietary carbohydrates and death.

As discussed in the intro of this book, jumping to conclusions from associations is often what leads medicine down the wrong path. This data does not chastise fat, protein, or carbohydrates, but merely reveals their association with different types of mortality in different countries. These associations may be surrogate markers for other factors that lead to excess mortality, but this is impossible to determine simply from the data available. Other variables may confound these findings. This remains a common shortcoming of epidemiologic studies, as they simply observe a snapshot in time of a group of people – no foregone conclusions can be made.

While many could use this data to boldly state that in order to live the longest, one must consume most of his or her calories from animal fat and avoid carbohydrates, Keys used it to chastise fat. His punishment was being featured on the cover of *Time* magazine in 1961, which showcased his data as the basis of the anti-fat movement within our country and the world. Interestingly enough, even Keys himself believed that cholesterol by itself had little to do with heart disease.

Rewinding several decades to the turn of the century, the human diet was primarily animal-based and was composed of a large percentage of animal meat and fat. Cooking products included saturated fats like bacon fat, also known as lard, beef fat, known as tallow, butter, and coconut oil, which is primarily saturated fat. Yet, the first myocardial infarction, or heart attack, was not even recorded until 1921. Nearly a decade later, in 1930, around 3,000 deaths within the U.S. were attributed to myocardial infarctions. Fast-forwarding three decades to 1960, this amount had risen to 500,000. Regardless of the data, dietary fat was labeled as an enemy of health, and efforts to avoid its consumption permeated the medical field for the next 50 years and continue to this day.

Data Ignored by Our Health Leaders

"In Framingham, Massachusetts, the more saturated fat one ate, the more cholesterol one ate, the more calories one ate, the lower people's serum cholesterol...we found that the people who ate the most cholesterol, ate the most saturated fat, ate the most calories weighed the least and were the most physically active."[23]
    –Dr. William Castelli,
    1992, director of the Framingham Health Study

In 1936, only several years after Anichkov's initial rabbit experiments, researchers at New York University attempted to assess whether cholesterol in humans correlated with atherosclerosis, the scientific term for damaged and clogged arteries. In order to accomplish this, Drs. Lande and Sperry performed extensive analyses via autopsies of healthy individuals who died abruptly. These were not the epidemiologic studies that Keys had performed but rather a direct look at cholesterol levels and atherosclerosis with the bodies to study.

Their experiments revealed no correlation between elevated levels of serum cholesterol, which is the amount of cholesterol contained within the blood, and clogged arteries. In fact, they only found that the prevalence of clogged arteries generally increased with age alone and not with increased serum cholesterol.[24] Lande and Sperry were not alone, as similar experiments on hundreds of autopsied bodies over the ensuing years confirmed these results.[25-28]

While rabbit studies were revealing an increase in arterial cholesterol accumulation from dietary fat and cholesterol, human studies were finding drastically different results. Such findings were not even considering the fact that the human body produces over three times more cholesterol than is present in the human diet. As a result, we attempted to look past rabbits.

Hundreds of millions of dollars were spent to further assess this relationship in humans, while simultaneously studies being performed in humans were revealing no correlation between blood cholesterol levels and atherosclerosis. To the surprise of many, this was occurring decades before the formation of the anti-fat guidelines. Newer studies had revealed that different subtypes of cholesterol may have differing effects on the rates of atherosclerosis, known as "good" cholesterol or HDL, and the "bad" cholesterol, known as LDL.[29] Even with this data, recent studies assessing aggressive lowering of the "bad" cholesterol with statins revealed no change in calcified plaques within arteries.[30] Recent randomized trials have revealed that "good" cholesterol was raised more often than not from *high-fat* diets.[31-37] The data and recommendations were in total disarray.

Clearly, medicine and science had no sound explanation as to which diet was optimal for reducing heart attack risk, and the question of which was best for reducing *overall* mortality, the most important factor, was being ignored. The practice of medicine should have realized this and avoided making any recommendations based on limited and faulty data. Unfortunately, the stage was set, and after the movement gained momentum, there was no stopping the anti-fat campaign.

While the war on fat aimed to decrease the consumption of this proposed deadly macronutrient in order to lower cholesterol levels, the necessity of fat and cholesterol within the diet and the physiologic necessity of cholesterol were forgotten. Low cholesterol has been associated with *increased* cancer risk,[16] individuals with high cholesterol have less risk of cancer,[38] and multiple studies have revealed that low cholesterol levels correlate with *increased* mortality.[17] Cholesterol, a necessity for life, was now the enemy.

GRAINS AND THE FOOD PYRAMID: FAT'S REPLACEMENT

"What right has the federal government to propose that the American people conduct a vast nutritional experiment, with themselves as subjects, on the strength of so very little evidence that it will do them any good?"
—Phil Handler,
president of the National Academy of Scientists

With the public lambasting of fat came the infamous food pyramid. When one food is eliminated from the diet, another food must replace it. In this case, it was carbohydrates, the same food that revealed an increase in overall mortality in Keys' data. The food pyramid and its praising of carbohydrates and grains has been the backbone of the dietary recommendations for the U.S. for nearly forty years. Riding on the coattails of the initial data blaming fat and cholesterol in the diet as the cause of coronary artery disease, fat soon was blamed for most modern diseases, including obesity.

The roots of the food pyramid can be traced back to 1977, less than two decades after Keys was on the cover of *Time* magazine. In the same year, George McGovern decided that the dietary habits of the citizens of the United States of America had to change, and they had to change drastically. While the transformation of the Standard American Diet can be traced to this time period, the history of grains is traced back much farther. However, while much older in origin than our modern dietary recommendations, the history of grains is rather miniscule when compared to the history of the human diet.

While humans are generally considered to be two to three million years old,[39] agriculture, or the domestication of plants, is a much more recent phenomena starting a mere 10,000 years ago.[40] At the end of the ice age, the glaciers receded exposing more land for grazing animals and plant life.[41] This allowed the spread and increase of both wild vegetation and plants that previously existed only in small quantities. Wild animals migrated from their homes to these new areas, and the human inhabitants gradually followed. Some areas, such as the Middle East, began to domesticate grains. While a controversial topic, prior to this time period, grains were likely only eaten in small amounts by humans, if at all.

The harvesting of crops first started around Western Asia in the Fertile Crescent and spread accordingly. For roughly two million years prior to the development of agriculture, the human diet consisted of food sources that were hunted and gathered.[42] Only recently have grains been considered the staple of the human diet.

Fast-forwarding several thousand years, George McGovern, from the grain-producing bastion of South Dakota, had little knowledge when it came to the science behind the effects of nutrition on the human body; nor should he have as a politician (McGovern was a long-time U.S. Senator and was the Democratic presidential nominee in 1972). However, these facts did not stand in the way of spearheading a movement to change the diet of the American people forever. He organized a committee to set up the guidelines, many of whom were his political colleagues, who were set to make millions of dollars off of the changes, which would financially support the main export of their state.

Under his guidance, the Dietary Goals of the United States were released, forever changing the face of the Standard American Diet as well as the rate of obesity.[16] The committee met and many who spoke at these committee meetings ferociously questioned McGovern. Some actually blamed carbohydrates for obesity. Such opposition was ignored. The committee passed its resolution with the following goals:

1. Increase carbohydrate consumption to account for approximately 55 to 60% of energy intake
2. Reduce overall fat consumption from 40 to 30% of energy intake
3. Reduce saturated fat consumption to account for 10% of total energy intake and balance that with polyunsaturated and monounsaturated fats, accounting for 10% of energy intake each
4. Reduce cholesterol consumption to about 300 mg/day
5. Reduce sugar consumption by about 40% to account for about 15% of total energy intake
6. Reduce salt consumption by 50-85% to about 3 g/day

The Nutritional Committee of the American Heart Association (AHA) refined these recommendations in 1982, aiming to reduce fat to less than ten percent of all consumed calories.

Interestingly, to support recommendations for such a drastic reduction in dietary fat, the AHA cited epidemiologic studies that actually showed no significant correlation between fat, cholesterol, and heart disease.[16] Two large studies that stand as the backbone of these recommendations were the Framingham Study and the Tecumseh Study.

The Framingham Study was a multimillion-dollar, massive study in Framingham, Massachusetts, that recruited 5,209 men and women from the ages of 30 to 62 in an effort to identify the dietary and lifestyle factors that contributed to cardiovascular disease. The physicians within the study performed extensive physical examinations and questionnaires to analyze lifestyle factors of each and every patient. This study was one of the largest undertakings in U.S. history; however, the results revealed no relationship between diet and cholesterol.[43] In fact, it was found that the more fat and overall calories each study participant ate, the lower the reading of his or her cholesterol.

The Tecumseh Study was a similar investigation assessing a large population in southeast Michigan over a 30-year period. Much like the Framingham Study, it found that serum cholesterol was not related to dietary consumption in its population. It did find that more obese individuals generally had higher cholesterol, but no relationship was seen with fat in the diet.[44] As obesity places an individual in a near constant state of inflammation, this once again may have been the body's physiologic response to inflammation by producing more cholesterol.

As a result, based on a lack of actual data, the U.S. government attempted to *guide* its population to good health. Unfortunately, it was based partly on nonexistent science and partly on faulty science. Once again, we ignored our history of a diet that for several million years was based on hunting and gathering, which likely included high amounts of fat and animal products, and replaced it with one that aimed to reduce this consumption to less than ten percent.

In doing so, this diet promoted the heavy consumption of grains, a relatively new food in the history of human beings. Under these new guidelines, Americans could guiltlessly consume over a staggering 300 grams of carbohydrates per day, and in the meantime expect to lose weight and lower their risk of heart disease. Over the next 30 years, the American people followed suit, increasing their carbohydrate intake while decreasing their dietary fat consumption.[4,6]

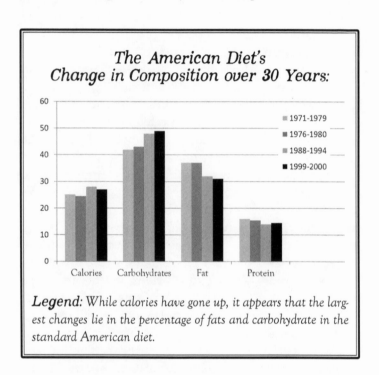

The American Diet's Change in Composition over 30 Years:

Legend: *While calories have gone up, it appears that the largest changes lie in the percentage of fats and carbohydrate in the standard American diet.*

The McGovern committee supplied the American people with a new dietary ideology in 1977, mostly in an effort to avoid heart disease and cancer. While the appropriate changes in the diet were actually made according to these recommendations, the American people watched as their rates of obesity skyrocketed over the next 30 years.[5] Yet, as is often the case in medical recommendation backed by little science but sustained through tradition, these recommendations continue to this day to perpetuate throughout the medical field and echo within the hallways of hospitals throughout the country.

Returning to George McGovern and the Dietary Goals of the United States, the lack of tangible science for the basis of such recommendations becomes clear as the U.S. healthcare system is being inundated by the results. It is now abundantly obvious what happens when we take data based on studies with rabbits, not humans, and foods that rabbits are unable to process, along with selective citation within Keys' research. Such adulteration of data and the human diet leaves little question as to why shortly after such recommendations were formed, obesity,[5] cardiovascular disease,[45] hypertension, diabetes,[46] and cancer[47] have all significantly risen in prevalence.

However, during the implementation of these recommendations over the past several decades and amid the discourse blaming fat and cholesterol in the diet as the cause of nearly every major health issue, many randomized studies have thoroughly assessed these recommendations. A plethora of studies have revealed that the data overwhelmingly points to carbohydrates as the opponent to weight loss and healthy arteries, and head-to-head comparisons of a low-fat and calorie-restricted diet have never shown to be superior to a high-fat diet.[31-37,48,49] In fact, in a majority of the studies, a high-fat diet unanimously results in health benefits.

In other words, the medical field advised the population to replace fat with a diet consisting mostly of carbohydrates, a food that has been repeatedly shown to lead to obesity. As a result, obesity and diabetes have reached unfathomable levels, and heart disease remains the number one killer of men and women.

However, the knowledge that carbohydrates, and not fat, lead to obesity and the metabolic diseases that follow, is not a new phenomenon. This has actually been known for thousands of years. While science was ignored to promote the low-fat agenda, once again history was also forgotten. As, Galen, the famous Roman physician of the emperor Marcus Aurelius, stated nearly twenty centuries ago:

> *"Thus the negros of the West Indies, and the Chinese slaves, sometimes acquire an enormous size during the sugar season, by drinking the cane-juice; the keepers of vineyards, who live on nothing but figs and grapes, become fat. The ladies of Tunis and Tripoli are fattened, to please the tastes of their lords, with farinaceous [starch] foods."*[50]

Or, as according to Count Leo Tolstoy, in his masterpiece *Anna Karenina*:

> *"He had no need to be in strict training, as he had very quickly been brought down to the required weight of one hundred and sixty pounds, but still he had to avoid gaining weight, and he avoided starchy foods and desserts."*[51]

Finally, in the words of Sir William Osler, considered one of the greatest physicians in the history of medicine and a founding father of Johns Hopkins Hospital:

> *"In the case of women who tend to grow stout after child-bearing or at the climacteric, in addition to systematic exercise, they should be told to avoid taking too much food, and particularly to reduce starches and sugars."*[52]

Similar Changes Are Seen in Animals from Altering Their Diet

A similar study of feeding animals large portions of food that they have not evolved to process has also taken place. Within the past several decades, grains have been fed to cows and other animals, replacing their natural diet of grass. Grass ferments in the rumen of cows, and then the cows digest the bacteria from this fermentation process. Feeding bison, beef, and other livestock grain feedlot is markedly different from the grass they are made to process, and it significantly affects their body composition.

In fact, feeding these animals grains causes the accumulation of fat throughout their carcass, and this method is now used to purposely fatten up livestock to increase the flavor of their meat.[53] This can be seen at the meat aisles of grocery stores where grain-fed meat is significantly more marbled with fat than grass-fed.

This simple experiment reveals what changes occur by altering an animal's natural diet, especially by basing the diet on grains. When the fat of these animals is assessed, it also contains much less amounts of healthy omega-3 fatty acids and cancer-fighting compounds like conjugated linoleic acid.[54] This simple change in the diet of these animals leads to fat accumulation and the forfeiture of natural cancer-fighting compounds.[55] As Americans have undergone a similar dietary experiment in the past century, it is no wonder that disease has skyrocketed in conjunction with these changes and it is naïve to assume the same issues would not happen in humans.

3

THE ADDICTIVE NATURE OF THESE RECOMMENDED FOODS

"I can now confidentially say that quantity of diet may be safely left to the natural appetite; and it is the quality only, which is essential to abate and cure corpulence."
   –William Banting,
      Letter on Corpulence Addressed to the Public, 1864

According to the Center for Disease Control, Americans may have increased their caloric intake during the past several decades. While exact calculations are difficult to perform, the medical field has frequently referred to this as the cause of obesity. Rarely are other factors considered, and there is little mention of the dietary recommendations that promote a food that leads to increased fat distribution within the body.

Also often forgotten is the fact that these recommendations demonize fat, a food that generally leaves one satiated after consumption. It is never mentioned that eating a diet solely based on carbohydrates creates severe hormonal imbalances that lead to weight gain.

While most data point to an increase in calories, few questions have been asked as to why this increase has occurred. Fast food and processed foods often take the brunt of the blame; however, rarely is the actual type of food consumed blamed for the resultant increase in calories. In fact, it is well established that when the human body encounters carbohydrates, a markedly different physiological response is experienced as opposed to when the body encounters foods heavy in protein or fat.

The physiologic response to carbohydrates actually leads to increased hunger and the consumption of more food.[56,57] While often described as simply the inability to eat just one potato chip or a single piece of bread prior to a meal, an underlying physiologic and biochemical response is actually to blame for this uncontrolled desire to consume more of these sugary and carbohydrate-rich foods.[58] In essence, we may have been prescribing addictive foods that increase the appetite and lead to obesity then blaming the individual for eating too much. Such a prescription would set up most people for failure and a lot of anxiety along the way.

Upon digging deeper, science has shown us that the body experiences a physiologic response to high amounts of sugar or carbohydrates present in bread, pasta, and other grains. As it encounters carbohydrates and grains, they are digested into simple sugars. In fact, eating a piece of white or wheat bread resembles little difference than a cupful of sugar once digested. As these sugars are dispersed into the blood stream, the body must act accordingly. If blood sugar becomes too high, it can quickly be fatal.

The body responds by secreting insulin, a hormone that

acts immediately to lower blood sugar by shuttling it from the blood and into the body's cells. Insulin also induces several other physiologic responses, including the stimulation of fat storage in adipose tissue. Conversely, when insulin is not present, the body burns fat to be used as a source of energy.[59] Therefore, it stands to reason that a diet with the goal of avoiding obesity would aim to reduce insulin spikes. Such a diet could not be composed of a preponderance of carbohydrates for the majority of the population.

When the body secretes large amounts of insulin into the bloodstream to lower blood sugar levels, these levels can frequently drop quicker than the body would like. As a result, hunger is once again stimulated in the body's effort to stabilize its blood glucose levels as it generally tries to avoid quick spikes and dips.[57] This ends in a vicious cycle of eating and hunger leading to weight gain and a society where obesity, a once unseen phenomenon, is now the norm.

This science of how our body deals with different foods was ignored by the committee that set the standard for the dietary habits of our society. Lost in the hyperbole was the fact that though fatty foods contain double the amount of calories as carbohydrates, they have little effect on insulin, and as a result, satisfy hunger[60] while carbohydrates stimulate it. Foods heavy in proteins satisfy hunger as well.[61,62]

Research has even shown that the larger the insulin response from food, the less these foods are able to satisfy hunger.[63] In other words, the larger the proportion of carbohydrates in a meal, the less satiating it is. As a result, it is no wonder that we created a society of overeaters. Remarkably, this was discussed in the literature as early as 1953, when it was found that individuals on calorically *unrestricted* diets lost weight as long as carbohydrates were restricted and replaced with fat.[64]

There are several other reasons for the addictive nature of carbohydrates and grains, including the fact that sugar and carbohydrates affect the same reward area of the brain where cocaine and other addictive drugs act.[65-68] Also, areas of the brain that control hunger and obesity are intimately related to carbohydrate intake through insulin. For instance, when an area of the brain known as the ventromedial hypothalamus is damaged, excessive amounts of insulin release ensues, as well as decreased insulin sensitivity, extreme appetite, and subsequent obesity.

It has been found that children with damage to this area after treatment for brain cancer experience excessive insulin release and intractable obesity. Yet, when insulin is blocked by a drug called octreotide, insulin levels drop, excessive food intake ceases, and they lose significant amounts of weight.[69]

Simply normalizing insulin levels changes several factors associated with obesity. Even in mice, it has been found that simply raising insulin levels alone results in obesity.[70] These experiments directly parallel those of our society, although on a smaller scale.

If dietary recommendations are currently favoring the consumption of more carbohydrates while eating less food overall, it becomes apparent that such recommendations are not only difficult to follow. Furthermore, they will likely create a psychological state of constant failure as these same patients are being told to bypass ingrained physiologic and hormonal response systems that are impossible to overcome.

Portion Control

A simple take on the dietary recommendations and over-consumption is to ask oneself how many times binging episodes occur when foods made entirely of fat and protein are consumed. Most people consider a salty steak delicious. How many times has consuming a steak lead to the consumption of another whole steak or two? How many times has the consumption of vegetables lathered with some grass-fed butter and salt become out of control?

Replace those vegetables with a piece of bread. How many times have you had "just one" piece of bread only to turn possessed and finish the entire basket? It is not a question of will power but rather one of physiology. We are unable to fight our bodily processes to overcome the addictive nature of these foods as we are hardwired to over-consume them. Fat and protein, however, are much more satiating, and studies have repeatedly shown that when individuals are placed on a low-carbohydrate diet without any restriction of calories, they naturally decrease their food intake because their hunger is satisfied.[62,71,72]

THE THERMODYNAMICS
OF EATING

*T*hough the exact inventor of the term "calorie" remains unknown, it appeared around 200 years ago, presenting itself in the literature somewhere between 1787 and 1824. It was originally used to quantify heat exchange in water and other materials, and its exact history remains unclear.[73] The caloric model gained momentum when Nicholas Clément furthered the science on the theory of steam engines in the early 1800s. Clément was a chemical engineer who worked extensively with heat transfer and followed the hypothesis that under the caloric model, heat, as a material, was always preserved.

Within the next century, the calorie model was eventually used to describe the amount of work needed to offset the force of gravity, to determine the least costly methods of providing livestock with nutrition through their feeds, and eventually to model the changes in heat from the different macronutrients in food. These experiments were initially performed to evaluate the economics of providing food macronutrients at a cheaper cost. These macronutrients included egg whites (proteins), sugars (carbohydrates), and fat. Eventually, a calorie was defined as the amount of work that could be performed from the energy content of foods, and the theory of daily energy intake and output based on calories was born.

Finally, the calorie was defined as the amount of heat needed to raise one kilogram of water by one degree Celsius. This energy of work included no physiologic variables and did not factor any hormonal or digestive effects. It was merely a measurement of heat and energy exchange.

The transition from the caloric models compiled by chemical engineers to present day food consumption has promoted the assumption that after food ingestion, it is either burned or stored, and this occurs equally with all foods based solely on calories. However, humans are not machines with simple input versus output mechanisms. We are diverse physiologic beings with millions of input and output mechanisms, hormones, genes, and innate processes that affect every minute aspect of energy usage, storage, and body character.

In fact, several hormones, including insulin, largely affect whether food is stored, burned, or converted to muscle versus fat, leaving the caloric model as an incredible feat for the 18th and 19th centuries, but it remains antiquated, outdated, and largely incorrect when extrapolated to humans and physique. When we factor in the composition of weight gain, i.e. muscle, which is desired by many, versus fat, which is desired by few, this model becomes even less relevant. This is in no way attempting to rewrite the laws of physics; however, it is clear that this model is more involved than its current state that simply eating more food equals gaining weight and vice versa. Unfortunately, this model remains ingrained in our current health model, as it has survived for well over a century with little advancement and does not appear to be at risk of extinction.

Along these lines, for many it will remain a simple equation of calories in versus calories out. If one consumes an extremely high amount of calories, weight gain will likely ensue, and conversely an extremely low calorie diet will likely leave someone without fat but also with low levels of muscle or energy. For example, Subway's "Jared" lost a significant amount of weight from starving himself with an extremely calorie-deprived diet over a long period of time. For many, including me, this is not sustainable for more than several days without extreme misery. For the remaining ninety-five percent of the population who is not subsiding on an extremely high or low caloric diet, other factors come into play.

According to the caloric model, if one consumes a diet of 2,000 calories of pure sugar versus a diet of 2,000 calories of fat and protein, body shape, weight, and energy output will remain the same. Followers of this model will naturally gravitate towards carbohydrates or proteins, as they only are composed of four calories per gram while fat is over double at nine calories per gram. However, science has revealed that this is not the case for several reasons.

Different foods absorbed within the body result in the release of different hormones and chemicals. As previously mentioned, significant amounts of carbohydrates within the diet cause a substantial release of insulin, which triggers fat storage. Conversely, when insulin levels are low, the body turns to the breakdown of fat for energy.

This fact alone is why, when compared in randomized scientific trials, the typical low-fat diet frequently recommended by our health leaders has never been shown to be superior to a low-carbohydrate, high-fat diet for weight loss; however, the low-carbohydrate diet has been shown to be superior in the vast majority of studies.[71] This is likely due to the significant drop in insulin that occurs from a low-carbohydrate diet, though the decrease in appetite that follows when limiting carbohydrates also clearly plays a part.

In the Presence of Insulin:

Dietary Carbohydrates & Fat ⟶ Bodyfat

Several studies have shown that a calorie is not a calorie when it comes to energy levels and body composition, and this is where the caloric model with regard to weight management and exercise begins to unravel. Human beings are physiologic specimens that like to stay in a state called *homeostasis*. In other words, the body will resist drastic changes by modifying its response to deviations from its normal state. For instance, if a person drastically reduces their dietary intake to lose weight, the body's metabolism will slow as well to compensate for this change and vice versa. This is why those on a calorically restricted diet often feel run down with little energy and are unable to exercise while those overeating have increased energy to engage in exercise and other activities. In fact, randomized studies show a significant decrease is resting metabolism in those that restrict calories.[74] This decrease in metabolism becomes even more prevalent in those that restrict calories and increase exercise.

This physiological slowing and hastening of the body's metabolism was the topic of recent research. In a recent study, three groups of individuals were placed on three separate diets, though they all consumed an equal number of calories.[75] The amount of fat, protein, and carbohydrates consumed were varied between the groups, leaving one group on a low-fat diet, another on a low-glycemic index diet (lower blood sugar raising), and the third group on a low-carbohydrate diet. Based on the caloric model, all three groups should have experienced the same changes in weight and metabolism; however, the results did not reveal these similarities. In fact, changes were markedly different between each diet group.

The typical metabolic and hormonal factors were analyzed in this study; but the unique aspect of this work was the measurement of resting energy expenditure, which represents the amount of calories required by the body during a day of non-activity. The higher the energy expenditure, the more the body burns throughout a day. Individuals that can eat large amounts of food without gaining weight are often labeled as having a high metabolism, and resting energy expenditure would be similar to this example. Therefore, in terms of achieving weight loss or maintaining decreased amounts of fat tissue, the higher the resting energy the better.

All diets in this study revealed a decrease in resting energy with weight loss. This is a common effect of dieting that makes it difficult for many to continue as metabolism slows and mood follows. This is homeostasis at work. In spite of this, the difference in the decrease in resting energy was significantly different between the diets. The decrease in resting energy was the *least* in the low-carbohydrate diet and *greatest* in the low-fat diet. In other words, the more carbohydrates one ate, the more one's metabolism slowed which makes fat loss substantially more difficult.

When Insulin is Minimally Present:

Bodyfat $\longrightarrow$ *Broken down* $\longrightarrow$ *Energy*

This data adds to the plethora of reasons why our nation is becoming obese at a rapid rate. Not only have Americans been instructed to eat appetite-stimulate foods that lead to overeating, they also have been put on a diet that significantly slows their metabolism, resulting in difficulty increasing activity or exercise, a clear recipe for disaster. These data basically revealed that weight loss on a low-carbohydrate diet, one that is the exact opposite of what the food pyramid and most health leaders recommend, leaves the dieter with a body that continues to burn more calories at rest. In other words, a low-carbohydrate diet leaves the body more metabolically demanding than the other diets.

Interestingly, this study also found that several metabolic variables were significantly different between the diets, further revealing that a calorie is not a calorie when it comes to the human body. For instance, leptin, the hormone that controls appetite and is associated with inflammation and cancer,[76-80] was found to be significantly lower in the low-carbohydrate dieters than the standard diet.

Insulin sensitivity, another major risk factor for cancer induction and recurrence,[81-85] was also lowest in the low-carbohydrate dieters. Serum HDL, or "good" cholesterol, was significantly higher in the low-carbohydrate diet versus the others, while serum triglycerides, which are associated with cardiovascular disease, stroke, and cancer,[28,86-88] were significantly less in the low-carbohydrate group versus the other two.

Finally, two inflammatory factors were assessed: plasminogen activator inhibitor 1, which has been found to be increased in cancer and is an indicator for cancer metastases (spread),[89] obesity, inflammation, and the metabolic syndrome,[90-92] and C-reactive protein (CRP), a marker of inflammation and has been correlated with poorer outcomes in cancer, stroke, depression, and cardiovascular disease.[93,94] Plasminogen activator inhibitor 1 had the largest drop in the low-carb group, while CRP dropped the most in the low-fat group. However, both were decreased in all groups, likely due to the weight loss. All markers of metabolic syndrome were improved in the low-carb diet; nonetheless, this has been shown many times before.[31,32,71,95-98]

Lastly, the fact that excess caloric consumption often gives individuals the energy to exercise more is misplaced in the minds of many health leaders, although it is well known by bodybuilders and athletes alike. The benefits of exercise are massive, from stopping osteoporosis[99] to reducing insulin levels,[100] and placing individuals on a strict calorie restricted diet often leaves them unable to exercise due to the severe slowing of their metabolism. In fact, bodybuilders often *increase* their calories while adjusting their macronutrient content to lose fat while maintaining or even gaining muscle.

Viewing weight loss as an in versus out equation is like putting less gas in your car to save money. The amount of gas you put in is not what leads to fuel efficiency. It is based on the machinery in the car, the engine mechanism, and the way the car is driven. The body, with its plethora of hormones and functions, is no different. In fact, sometimes putting in higher-grade fuel makes it run more efficiently, and the same happens in weight loss. It is about the quality of the fuel used and the engine that is burning it.

Do Some Foods Favor Muscle versus Fat Gain?

"Protein intake predicted the increase in lean body mass, but not the change in fat storage."
—Dr. George Bray,
Professor, Pennington Biomedical Research Center

Many have questioned the importance of the composition of food as opposed to calories to enable the body to burn fat and build muscle. It has been questioned whether varying dietary carbohydrates or protein alone could lead to greater fat loss. While often weight loss or weight gain is viewed as the only variable of importance in dieting, realistically the goal is to decrease fat while maintaining or even increasing muscle mass.

As a result, another study was undertaken to assess the effect of the protein content of food on weight gain, body composition, and energy expenditure.[101] In this study, patients were placed in the metabolic ward of the hospital and asked to consume an *extra* 954 calories per day in an attempt to gain weight. They were placed into three groups and the diets were as follows:

1. Low-protein diet: 6% of energy from protein, 52% from fat, and 42% from carbs
2. Normal protein diet: 15% of energy from protein, 44% from fat, and 41% from carbs
3. High-protein diet: 26% of energy from protein, 33% from fat, and 41% from carbs

Unfortunately, all groups were placed on a high carbohydrate diet, limiting the assessment of carbohydrate modification. As expected, all groups gained weight; however the first group consuming the lower amount of protein and higher amount of fat gained about seven pounds, while the other groups gained thirteen pounds. Yet, when taking a closer look, lean body mass, which is composed of mostly muscle, decreased in the low protein group by two pounds, while the higher protein groups experienced an increase in muscle mass by over six pounds. When looking at the increase in fat mass in both groups, all three gained about seven pounds. Basically, everyone put on weight, with all groups gaining the same amount of body fat, but the high protein group gaining nearly triple the amount of lean muscle mass.

Also, similarly to the previous study, overeating in the higher protein groups led to a significant increase in resting energy as well as increased energy expenditure. In other words, overeating increased this group's metabolism, providing them with more energy to exercise and build more muscle. Homeostasis, the process by which the body aims to remain in a steady state, once again led to these changes; therefore if one were to eat more, in this case protein, metabolism increases to enable the body to burn the extra calories and vice versa. However, the increase is clearly different based upon the different type of foods consumed. Once again, a calorie is not necessarily a calorie when it comes to the body, diet, and exercise.

THE NON-NUTRIENT
AND ANTI-NUTRIENT
"BENEFITS" OF GRAINS

While the food pyramid was clearly off of the mark in chastising fats and recommending appetite-stimulating, fat-producing carbohydrates, an even larger mistake may have been the types of carbohydrates recommended. The bulk of these recommendations endorsed bread, cereal, pasta, and grains – six to eleven servings per day to be exact. While this massive amount of bread and pasta will lead to weight gain for most, there are several other problems with such a recommendation.

Just as animals have sharp teeth and claws as a defense mechanism to ward off prey, it appears that plants also contain defense mechanisms, especially grains. Plants and animals need to reproduce and survive, and both employ methods to ensure this occurs. While the weapons of defense are more obvious in animals, grains have biochemical weapons that physiologically disrupt their prey, partially in an effort to make the prey avoid them in the future and partially in an effort to ensure they can survive and reproduce.

When these food sources are eaten, they are often indigestible and therefore are passed through the body, ending up in the stool for future germination. During their path, these food sources create havoc by causing trauma to the lining of the intestines and stimulating an inflammatory reaction. It is clearly advantageous for the offspring of a plant to be able to travel through the intestines, pulling cellular debris and undigested nutrients with it along the way ending up in a pile of fertilizer. Just as humans and animals have developed techniques to survive, so have plants and grains.

Grains are often touted as a rich source of fiber and nutrients, like vitamin B, iron, magnesium, selenium, and folic acid. Most grains are actually refined, which involves the mechanical removal of the germ or bran. This is often accomplished through bleaching the grains, which strips them of their nutrients, leaving an insulin-raising carbohydrate source not much different biologically from pure table sugar. They are then "enriched" with the nutrients listed above which basically means that factory produced nutrients and vitamins are added back to them. Whole grains are often considered healthy while refined grains are not. Yet, randomized studies reveal there may be little difference in regards to their effect on insulin and other metabolic factors.[102]

When comparing grains with other sources of foods with less insulin-raising effects, like leafy green vegetables and animal fat and protein, grains are significantly less nutrient-dense. In other words, one gets significantly more nutrients with much less insulin secreted within the body with non-grain sources. As a result, the need for vitamins, nutrients, energy, and hunger satisfaction is much more easily accomplished with non-grain food types.

Grains also appear to have anti-nutrients, possibly even

more detrimental to our health, which are proteins that bind to necessary vitamins and nutrients and leave them unable to be digested and absorbed. Grains also appear to damage the lining of our gastrointestinal tract causing digestion issues. As a result, grains often pass through our system, accompanied with nutrients, vitamins, cellular debris, and stool – the perfect recipe for plant survival. A summary of these anti-nutrients is described by three main points below.

Phytic Acid

Phytic acid is the storage form of phosphorus in many plants, including legumes, nuts, seeds, and grains. It is also found in leafy green vegetables but in considerably smaller amounts. While it does have some antioxidant effects like most fruits and vegetables, it has many negative aspects that fruits and vegetables do not.

Phytic acid, also known as phytate, is indigestible when consumed by humans, and as it passes through the gastrointestinal tract undigested, it binds to several nutrients and prohibits their absorption into the body. These vital nutrients include calcium, magnesium, zinc, vitamin B3, and iron. While grains may contain a moderate amount of iron, niacin, and magnesium, these benefits are minimized as the phytic acid content within the grains limits the absorption of these nutrients.

The detrimental effect of phytates is not only limited to impairing the direct absorption of vitamins and minerals through chelation (binding). They also appear to inhibit and even inactivate several enzymes that are necessary to digest proteins, carbohydrates, and even fats, further impairing the absorption of nutrients.[103] These unabsorbed phytates are eventually passed into the environment, where they are known to pollute the soil and drinking water.[104]

Lectin

Beans, seeds, some nuts, and most grains contain large amounts of lectin, a complex protein that also causes several physiologic reactions when consumed. Much like pollens or other allergens, lectin causes an immunologic and antigenic reaction within the body. The immune response triggered by lectin can result in autoimmune diseases, which occur when extreme or repetitive stimulation of the immune system leads to a sustained response, as seen in diseases like rheumatoid arthritis or lupus.[105]

Similar to the ability of phytates to interact with the absorption of nutrients within our intestinal lining, lectin has been also shown to damage intestinal cells and even inhibit their ability to repair themselves.[106] This damage results in what has been coined a "leaky gut," or basically a damaged intestinal or gut lining that can allow bacteria, infectious elements, and toxins through its lining into the bloodstream. These detrimental effects are of vital importance as the gut lining is one of the body's first and main defenses against foreign pathogens found in food and the environment.

Interestingly, much like phytates, lectin is likely a defense mechanism for plants to deter predators from consuming them. Lectins can also bind to kidney cells and damage them, leading to leakage of protein in the urine. They also act as antigens and bind to receptors on pancreatic cells, potentially leading to diabetes.[107]

Much like the sugar fructose, lectin has been shown to lead to leptin resistance. Leptin is the chemical within our body that affects many physiologic functions, including suppressing appetite. Leptin resistance results in increased appetite and obesity,[78] and lectin is one of the many aspects of grains that leads to overeating. Again, recommending foods that lead to overeating is a massive cause of the current obesity crisis.

Finally and most importantly, lectin is able to travel throughout the body, bind to receptors on cells that are potentially harmful, and activate them. These receptors include the insulin receptor and epidermal growth factor receptor (EGFR),[108] both of which have been heavily implicated in cancer and are also recent targets of many novel therapeutic cancer drugs.[109,110] They have also been shown to initiate mitogenesis,[111] which is the process of cell division. Over-stimulation of mitogenesis is a potential cause of cancer.

Due to many of these aspects of lectin, it is also used in biochemical warfare. A part of the highly toxic poison, ricin is a lectin, which binds to the cell surface and is absorbed in the cell inhibiting its function and causing death. Lectins are in beans, peanuts, and other legumes, not just cereals and grains, and dairy from cows fed grains also have higher amounts as the lectins are passed from their feed.

Gluten

Gluten is possibly the most famous of the toxins found in grains. It is a protein composed of gliaden and glutelin and is found in many grains, including barley, rye, and wheat. Wheat, the backbone of the food pyramid, contains significant amounts of gluten. Gluten is also frequently added to imitation meats and processed foods and can even be found in ice cream and ketchup, as it is used as a stabilizing agent. Gluten gives dough its rubbery texture and the ability to rise and form a spongy consistency during baking, ultimately forming bread.

Similar to phytic acid and lectin, gluten causes an inflammatory and immune reaction within the body when consumed. Gluten also results in severe damage to the cells along the lining of the intestinal tract.[112] This once again results in a "leaky gut," allowing the entrance of foreign invaders when the lining of the intestines becomes increasingly permeable after gluten contact.[113] This increased permeability also attracts inflammatory cells and stimulates damaging cytokine production.[114]

Celiac disease, a condition defined as severe intolerance to gluten with resulting gastrointestinal, psychological, and other side effects from gluten within the diet, is diagnosed in around one percent of the population. In these individuals, the consumption of gluten results in severe inflammatory reactions and autoimmune disease ensues, as the body begins to attack the gluten and itself.[115,116]

While an area of current controversy, newer data is revealing that one does not have to suffer from a diagnosis of celiac disease to suffer from the intolerance of gluten.[117] Some have even questioned whether all individuals are gluten sensitive to varying degrees, though this is controversial and unanswered in the current data. However, individuals with known gluten sensitivity can also experience immunologic attacks on their nervous system, resulting in cerebellar ataxia (damage to the brain) and peripheral neuropathy (damage to the nerves in the extremities).[118] The conditions present as difficulty walking, pain, numbness, tingling, and decreased ability to perform fine motor function in the extremities.[119] Gluten sensitivity has even been shown to cause seizures, epilepsy,[120] and schizophrenia.[121] The detrimental effects of consuming foods that result in overstimulation of the immune system become quite obvious when seen in celiac patients.

Studies have shown that a myriad of conditions can be improved with the removal of gluten from the diet. Patients with dermatitis herpetiformis, a disease causing red and painful skin lesions, are often cured when placed on a gluten-free diet.[122] Dermatitis herpetiformis is an autoimmune disease where the body begins to attack itself after repeated immune system stimulation by the toxins in grains. Similarly, patients with Crohn's disease have also been found to go into remission when wheat is eliminated from the diet.[123]

Just as gluten causes the neurological disorders listed above, recently there has been data pointing towards gluten as partly responsible for the rise in autism. In fact, removing gluten from the diet has been shown in clinical trials to be a treatment for autism.[124] Gluten sparks an autoimmune reaction that may attack brain cells, and this is especially crucial for young children as their brains are developing at this life stage. Interestingly, the rise in autism has correlated with the rise in grain consumption; however, the recent change in the diagnosis criteria for autism makes any concrete conclusions difficult.[125]

While we cannot know for sure if grain and gluten consumption *causes* autism, we can study children already diagnosed with autism to assess if there is any improvement when they are removed. Recent studies reveal that when autistic children have gluten removed from their diet, they experience a significant improvement in a number of behavioral aspects.[126] These changes are not only seen clinically, but specialized imaging called SPECT scans, which measure metabolic activity of cells and tissues within the body, reveal changes in brain function with the removal of gluten from the diet.

One study in a patient with undiagnosed and untreated gluten intolerance and psychiatric symptoms revealed decreased activity in the frontal lobe of the brain. A functioning frontal lobe allows individuals to differentiate between good and bad, suppress socially unacceptable behaviors, and retain long-term memories. The frontal lobe in essence enables individuals to acclimate to social situations, a task often absent or altered in those with autism. However, when all gluten is removed from the diet, their symptoms resolved and repeat SPECT scans revealed a disappearance of the brain dysfunction.[127]

Like phytates and lectin, gluten consumption can result in deficiencies in other vitamins and minerals and has been shown to cause selenium deficiency, which can lead to thyroid damage. Coincidently, gluten causes the release of harmful inflammatory chemicals that also damage the thyroid.[128]

On a side note, compounds similar to gluten, called saponins, are found in some grains. Similar to lectins, they are a protective chemical for the plants that contain them, as they cause adverse reactions in their predators when consumed.[129] They have even been used with vaccines to allow modified viruses to enter the system much easier through the gut. While they do not appear to bind to receptors in the GI tract, they directly promote leaky gut syndrome, allowing pathogens to directly enter the blood stream and promote a state of inflammation.[130] The constant state of inflammation produced by these so-called healthy foods becomes worrisome when, as discussed previously, more and more data is pointing to inflammation as the main culprit of heart disease and even cancer.

Interestingly, while gluten has received much attention in the media for all of the problems it causes, lectins and phytic acids are possibly even more harmful. A final component of grains is a substance called lipopolysaccharide (LPS). LPS is a component of the outer surface of bacteria and is what is known as an endotoxin. When encountered in humans, it stimulates a potent inflammatory response by the immune system. In fact, it is so potent that even a small amount can result in septic shock, an often fatal event. While mice and other rodents appear to be somewhat resilient to LPS, humans are exquisitely sensitive to its detrimental effects.[131]

Studies in animals reveal that when they are fed a diet of grains, like wheat and barley, they experience a translocation of LPS from the gastrointestinal tract and into the circulatory system, resulting in significant inflammation.[132] This is likely why data in humans reveal that switching to a diet of whole grains results in increased levels of oxidized LDL, or so called "bad cholesterol,"[133] the same culprit that causes cardiovascular disease, as previously discussed.

While data for heart disease varies based upon the source, hospital admissions for heart disease continue to increase. Due to the advancement of medicine, mortality from heart disease appears to be decreasing. Although, if the American people have been decreasing the amount of heart disease-causing fat they consume and replacing it with "heart healthy" grains, then why is heart disease not dropping drastically?

Just as scientists found in the rabbits mentioned above, cholesterol and fat were not necessarily causing the heart disease but rather offsetting the inflammation. Promoting foods like grains that allow toxic substances to cross into the blood supply, igniting a cascade of inflammation, is likely fueling the process of heart disease. Unfortunately, a byproduct of this increase in heart disease via inflammation may also be increasing rates of cancer, diabetes, and several other chronic diseases. While it is unclear if it is necessary to completely remove all grains from the diet, the health detriment of basing an entire diet on grains is quite obvious.

PART TWO

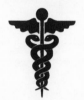

THE RECALL ON FAT
AND ITS ADVANTAGES

*"We are lucky to still be alive. We ate all
the bad foods during our younger years
– lard, butter, and fatty cuts of meat. In
fact, we always saved the fat for our
fathers, as it was considered the best
part of the meal."*
    —*Rose and John Reichl, **96** years old,
    and Rose, 92*

THE CHEMISTRY OF
FATS AND OILS

*A*fter several decades of havoc from the new dietary recommendations, some physicians and scientists started to notice the destruction that these dietary changes were creating. Eventually, the target was slowly moved from all fats to only saturated fats. It stood to reason that polyunsaturated fats and vegetable oils, which are liquid at room temperature, are healthy fats that will not accumulate within the arteries, leading to disease.

Saturated fats like butter, coconut oil, or bacon fat, on the other hand, are solid at room temperature and were thought to clearly be the culprit behind the diseased state of our nation. Thus, polyunsaturated fats and vegetable oils were coined as "heart healthy" and were introduced into the diet as salad dressings and cooking agents.

However, before the health effects of vegetable oils and polyunsaturated fats are assessed, their chemistry must be considered as the two are intimately related.

While saturated fats are solid at room temperature, polyunsaturated oils remain liquid, allowing many to conclude that saturated fat can accumulate within the arteries, while polyunsaturated fats, like vegetable oil, can easily pass through. Just like the initial thought that fat in the diet led to fat accumulation within the body, such simplistic thinking, while reasonable, is incorrect.

Saturated fat remains solid at room temperature due to its molecular structure, which is so stable that the melting point is higher than room temperature. Thus coconut oil stays solidified in the jar when placed at room temperature or if kept in the refrigerator. However, unsaturated fats are far less molecularly stable and become liquid at room temperature. This structural difference is the result of the number of carbon atoms on the backbone of the fat that are unbound with hydrogen. Basically, the more unbound carbons, the more unsaturated a fat is and the higher likelihood that it will remain liquid at room temperature.

Oil, with few exceptions, is essentially a fat that is liquid at room temperature. Coconut oil, for example, is usually solid at room temperature due to its high melting point. For instance, if ice melted at 78 degrees instead of 32, it would often remain solid at room temperature. While many people assume that all oil is made up of unsaturated fatty acids, coconut, palm, and several other oils are actually partially composed of saturated fat.

Saturated Fat

Monounsaturated fats have a single unsaturated site which means that there is a double bond between two carbons and each of these carbon atoms do not have hydrogen atoms bound to them (the arrows below). Olive oil is mostly mono-unsaturated, but unlike its vegetable oil cousins, it is made by an entirely different process.

Monounsaturated Fat

Polyunsaturated fats have many free and unsaturated carbon atoms on their backbone. This also leaves them less structurally sound and liquid at room temperature.

Polyunsaturated Fat

Monounsaturated fatty acids are different from polyunsaturated fatty acids (PUFAs) in that they only have one double bonded pair of carbon atoms on their backbone. Because these carbons are unbound, they are therefore unprotected and can be attacked by free radicals and become oxidized. This oxidized fatty acid can then travel along and cause damage in a remote area of the body such as in an artery. Polyunsaturated fats, on the other hand, have many sites that can be attacked by free radicals, increasing the potential risk of damage from oxidation.

A simple way to conceptualize this is to consider that all fats have a chain of carbon atoms as their backbone. Similar to a spine, there is a whole chain of these carbon atoms that can be bound or unbound by a hydrogen atom. Each carbon atom is a vertebra, and if the vertebra has a hydrogen atom attached, there is less room for a free radical to enter and attack. As a result, the free radical passes by, looking for an unprotected and unbound vertebra.

Along these lines, saturated fats have no unexposed weak points for this roaming free radical to attack, while unsaturated fats have many. This becomes extremely important when these oils are placed under heat for cooking, as they interact with many free radicals during the cooking process.

Out with Saturated Cooking Fats

During its entrance and rise in popularity within American society, McDonald's fast food hamburger chain was famous for its golden French fries. These fries were cooked in tallow, lard, and palm oil. Tallow, which is beef fat, and lard, which is pork fat, along with palm oil, contain significant amounts of saturated fat. While lard and tallow are solid at room temperature, they quickly melt in a heated pan or fryer. However, recently nearly all fast food restaurants have replaced these cooking oils with peanut and canola oil, as well as a plethora of other polyunsaturated vegetable oils that are often advertised as "heart healthy."

The advent of these oils into the fast food business can be traced back to the 1980s, when the Center for Science in the

Public Interest (CSPI) led an assault on McDonald's for using lard and saturated fats to cook its fries. These saturated fats were labeled as extremely damaging to heath in a public campaign, and thus they were replaced. There was little evidence to support such claims; yet, a smear campaign was damaging enough to force McDonald's to make the switch from cooking with saturated fats. New cooking oils like Crisco and margarine, which were composed of partially hydrogenated fats known as trans-fats, entered the fast food scene. These fats are manufactured to mimic the properties of saturated fats by remaining solid at room temperature, but they are initially composed of unsaturated fats. At the time, the CSPI even labeled Burger King's switch to partially hydrogenated oil as "a great boon to American's arteries."

This maligning of saturated fats ushered in the usage of partially hydrogenated oils, and the spread of trans-fats throughout our society followed.[134] Several decades later, the U.S. is experiencing an aggressive campaign to remove trans-fats from our kitchens and restaurants, as recent studies have revealed the harmful nature of these fats. Recent data have shown that replacing saturated fats with trans-fats decreases HDL, known as the "good" cholesterol that helps remove the accumulation of "bad" cholesterol within the arteries.

Further studies have revealed that replacing saturated fat with trans-fats can lead to blood vessel damage, possibly causing the initial insult that leads to atherosclerosis.[135] Most worrisome, the consumption of trans-fats elevates several inflammatory pathways like IL-6 and CRP, which are known to damage the lining of the arteries and severely stress the body.[136] This event signified the change in beliefs toward fat and health and began the journey down the wrong pathway.

In with Vegetable Oils

Just as saturated fats were wrongly replaced with pro-inflammatory trans-fats, leading to increased health risks, this trend eventually continued with the segue from saturated fats to polyunsaturated vegetable oils. The health benefits of these oils seemed obvious as they were made from "heart-healthy" vegetables and served to replace the artery-clogging saturated fats and unhealthy factory produced trans-fats.

While many praise the health benefits of vegetables oils, few even know how vegetable oils are actually produced since many of the vegetables used to make these oils actually contain little to no fat or oil. In fact, while consuming trans-fats is clearly a health risk, some studies in mice have shown that switching to corn oil, a common vegetable oil, actually results in increased colon cancer in comparison to trans-fats. Shockingly, corn and other vegetable oils high in linoleic acid are often used in animal studies to cause cancer.[137,138] When polyunsaturated fats replaced saturated fats in a randomized controlled trial in humans, the rates of cancer actually rose and started to accelerate drastically during the time that the trial was closed.[139] Switching to vegetable oils furthered the U.S. down this wrong pathway.

THE INDUSTRIAL PROCESS OF CREATING VEGETABLE OILS: CHEMICAL REFINEMENT

*C*onverting a vegetable or plant-based substance into oil is a complicated chemical process. The oil is not simply squeezed out of the vegetable, as many would believe. The process generally begins with a nut, seed, or polyunsaturated fat source, which, as described above, has many free carbons that are defenseless against heat damage and free radical attack. The final product is one of the many common vegetable oils, including:

1. Rapeseed oil, also known as Canola oil
2. Peanut oil
3. Soybean oil
4. Sunflower oil
5. Corn oil
6. Grapeseed oil

Intense chemical and mechanical manipulation of the vegetable source is required during production, which removes
many of the natural elements and nutrients within these
sources. The step-by-step process is below.

Step 1: Pressing

The first step in refinement involves extracting the small
amount of oil from the chosen plant-based source. This usually involves gathering seeds that are often genetically engi-
neered to be immune to pesticides, crushing them, heating
them to high temperatures, pressing them, and finally, bath-
ing them in a hexane bath with other solvents made from
crude petroleum.

The oil is then separated from the seed residue and phosphate is added. The residue that is collected is often used as
animal feed. This step takes the already defenseless polyunsaturated fat and further damages it through thermal, chemical,
and physical manipulation, introducing many free radicals
into its unprotected carbon backbone.

Step 2: Neutralization, Bleaching, and Deodorization

The oxidized damage from the initial step in this process
leaves the oil with a foul odor and unwanted color. This substance is then bleached to remove the unwanted color. The
final process involves steaming the oils with extremely high
temperatures, often over 500° F, in order to remove residual
substances that may cause an unwanted taste or odor. This
step is referred to as deodorization.

Deodorization and the high heat with which the oil encounters during steaming may be most damaging, as it severely weakens the fatty acids, leaving it further structurally
impaired and oxidized by the heavy barrage of free radicals

that it encounters. Also, many refined vegetable oils also contain added butylated hydroxytoluene (BHT) and butylated hydroxyanisole (BHA),[140] both of which have been shown to cause bladder and thyroid cancer in animals.[141]

The Final Product:

While the health implications are quite obvious just from the process of making vegetable oil, further detriments occur during storage. The destruction of the backbone of the oil leaves it oxidized and defenseless against future free radical damage during storage and cooking.

As a result, the shelf life of vegetable oil is extremely short, and it can often go rancid after only six months of storage time. Even unrefined olive oil, which is produced by different methods than those described above, goes rancid after six months. Coconut oil, on the other hand, can effectively fight off free radical damage during storage for a year or two, as it is high in saturated fat. Walnut and sesame oil can go rancid in as little as two months.

A final issue throughout the processing of vegetable oils is the destruction of antioxidants present within the oils that serve as a defense against free radical damage. This process destroys antioxidants, like vitamin E. Oil that is not produced by this process, such as coconut, olive, and macadamia nut oil, avoids the destruction of their antioxidants and vitamins. In fact when macadamia nuts, which contain an ample amount of antioxidants,[142] are made into oil, it remains relatively full of antioxidants.[143]

Note that virgin olive oil is produced through more physical means and not the chemical treatment described above. However, both refined olive oil and pomace oil (a type of olive oil) undergo chemical treatment. Although unrefined, virgin, and organic coconut oil avoid chemical processing as well, one can also still find some chemically altered coconut oil, which is known as RBD (refined, bleached, and deodorized).

The process of producing vegetable oils through neutralization, bleaching, and deodorizing is clearly unnatural and likely unsafe. The final chemical product of vegetable oil quickly goes rancid with its short shelf life and is defenseless against free radical attack. Adding to insult is the fact that it is stripped of healthy antioxidants and often contains cancerous chemicals and compounds.

Common Sources of Monounsaturated Fat
(with percentages of monounsaturated fat):

1. Macadamia oil: 85%
2. Olive oil: 75%
3. Avocado oil: 70%
4. Tallow (beef fat): 50%
5. Lard (pork fat): 40%

Vegetable Oils:

1. Rapeseed oil
2. Canola oil
3. Peanut oil
4. Soybean oil
5. Sunflower oil
6. Corn oil
7. Safflower oil
8. Grape seed oil
9. Sesame Oil

Most Structurally Sound Cooking Oils/Fats:

1. Macadamia oil
2. Coconut oil
3. Avocado oil
4. Olive oil (to garnish, not necessarily cook)
5. Grass-fed butter
6. Tallow or lard

CONJUGATED LINOLEIC ACID – THE FORGOTTEN ALLY IN THE BATTLE AGAINST BEEF

"Animal fat, which has been maligned for so long, may actually contribute a potent therapeutic component to our diet."[144]
–David Kritchevsky, Ph.D.,
former president of the American Society
of Nutritional Sciences

*L*ost in the crusade against fat were its many health benefits. Cholesterol and saturated fats are required for hormone production and the body's cells are lined with fat as a protective barrier. Not only are some fatty foods nutrient-dense, but also many contain fat-soluble vitamins and nutrients that are vital for health.

Conjugated linoleic acid (CLA) is formed from a simple change in the geometric structure of linoleic acid, an unsaturated fat commonly found in many foods. While CLA has a structure similar to that of linoleic acid, the manner in which each affects the body is strikingly different. CLA is found in the fat of ruminant animal meat and milk, including cheese, butter, and dairy.[145]

Ruminant animals, like cows, are those that have a rumen in their gastrointestinal tract. The rumen is where grass remains after it is eaten. As the grass sits within the rumen, it begins to ferment and bacteria from the rumen consume these fermented remains.[146] The intestines of the cows then basically consume the bacteria for nourishment.

Humans, on the other hand, do not possess a rumen and cannot process grass and cellulose as it simply passes through undigested. The largest amounts of CLA can be found in beef, lamb, butter, and cream, and lesser amounts are found in in turkey and veal. However, these animals must be fed grass, which is their natural diet. In the past several decades, the grass diet of cows has been replaced with grains, corn, and soy. These foreign sources of food create an acidic environment within the rumen, which does not allow for sufficient bacterial growth and significantly reduces the amount of CLA that is synthesized in these animals. CLA content in fish is minimal, and there are near-negligible amounts in vegetable oils.

CLA and Cancer

CLA had an undeniable connection with cancer from the onset of its discovery. It was originally discovered when scientists were attempting to cause cancer by creating heterocyclic amines and hydrocarbons. These substances are formed in burnt meat and have been shown to result in cancer in laboratory studies.[144,147] Interestingly, as the scientists were frying the beef, they uncovered a new substance that was eventually called conjugated linoleic acid. The study turned into one of many experiments where creating a villain produces a hero, as it was found that the CLA actually stopped the progression of normal cells to cancer, a process known as mutagenesis. It was hard for many to believe that a substance from fried beef could help fight cancer, but the results showed otherwise.

Many studies followed, and most exposed mice and rats to toxic chemicals called carcinogens. Carcinogens lead to high rates of cancer induction, and studies attempted to assess the ability of CLA to impede the development of cancer. The animals were given different diet regimens containing CLA at varying time points, including prior to exposure to toxic chemicals, during exposure, or afterwards. The studies uniformly revealed dramatic decreases in cancer incidence. Human cell lines in laboratory studies have confirmed these results, also revealing a decrease in cancer occurrence. Large human trials remain undone, but many hope that this will change as more of the scientific community begins to realize the importance of diet and nutrition in cancer care.[148]

For example, in one of the studies, mice were fed different amounts of CLA and exposed to a cancer-causing or carcinogenic chemical that causes breast cancer. The carcinogen led to cancer in eighty percent of the mice on a normal diet while this amount was halved in those mice consuming CLA.[149] Other studies have shown that the benefits of CLA reach beyond halting cancer induction as studies in mice with prostate cancer have revealed a reduction in the occurrence of cancer spread, known as metastases.

In a similar study, mice with cancer were either given linoleic acid or CLA. Cancer metastases occurred in nearly all mice fed the linoleic acid, while only ten percent of those fed CLA experienced spread of their cancer.[150] Other studies compared CLA, linoleic acid, and olive oil. While olive oil had no effect on cancer induction, linoleic acid promoted it, and CLA was successful in fighting cancer.[151]

Linoleic Acid

Linoleic acid is a fatty acid found in large proportions in vegetable oils, such as walnut, sesame, and canola oil. Twenty percent of chicken fat is made up of this fatty acid, and egg yolks contain fifteen percent.[152] It is found in minimal amounts in butter, macadamia oil, and coconut oil. Contrary to CLA, it has been shown to enhance the occurrence of cancer in animal studies.[153] Corn oil, heavy in linoleic acid, is often used in experiments to *cause* high levels of cancer in animals. Even when linoleic acid has been given as a carcinogen, CLA can overcome this mutagenic effect of vegetable oils and limit cancer formation.[149]

Can Eating More Beef Help Fight Breast Cancer?

CLA appears to have an important relationship with all types of cancer; however, breast cancer may be most significant. While CLA has been shown to decrease skin, liver, and colon cancer in animal studies, results with breast cancer have been the most remarkable. Much like the mouse studies discussed above, CLA was successful in stopping chemically-induced breast cancer. It was also found that when animals were fed CLA, it was incorporated into their fatty breast tissue.

In other words, in response to a substance that may protect cells from cancer, the body appears to store CLA in its fat tissue in an effort to help defend against cancer. In the field of cancer medicine, methods to localize breast cancer treatment are constantly undertaken; yet, it appears that the body may engage in this naturally by placing a cancer-fighting substance directly within the breasts. Studies also reveal that breast cancer cells may extract CLA directly from the diet or local environment leading to their death.[149] As a side note, CLA is also incorporated into the brain and liver and likely serves to protect these areas from cancer as well.

Since CLA has been shown to fight cancer in animal studies, its placement in breast tissue leads to the logical conclusion that it would decrease the risk of breast cancer, and population studies support this theory. A recent study in a group of Finnish women analyzed dietary CLA and blood levels of CLA and found that dietary CLA was significantly associated with a decreased risk of breast cancer.[154]

Is CLA an Antioxidant?

Reducing inflammation in the body likely reduces the risk of cancer.[155] On a daily basis the body receives nearly constant insult from free radicals, stress, and trauma, resulting in inflammation, oxidation, and cell damage. This damage may result from sources that are impossible to avoid, such as chemicals and toxins ubiquitous to our environment or from free radicals within our diet. Regardless of the source, the human body is constantly bombarded with potential threats. As a result, it must constantly build up its arsenal to help fight this bombardment. Antioxidants play a large part in this as they help to fight and fix the oxidation that occurs when a free radical attacks; thus, the term *anti-oxidant*.

Just as fats and oils can be oxidized from cooking and storage, this oxidation can be passed onto the body to cause damage. As discussed previously, oxidized fat is likely a major culprit responsible for atherosclerosis and clogged arteries, not fat alone. A continuation in the theme of rabbit studies and cholesterol has revealed that if they are fed a diet rich in fat and cholesterol, similar to Anichkov's initial experiments, but supplemented with CLA, atherosclerosis is reversed by up to fifty percent.[156] Interestingly, in this study, cholesterol numbers remained unchanged as rates of atherosclerosis were decreased.

Improved Glucose Tolerance, Weight Loss, and Increased Lean Mass from CLA

CLA ingestion also reduces levels of omega-6 fatty acids in rat tissue while increasing levels of omega-3 fatty acids. As will be discussed further below, elevated levels of omega-6 fatty acids are inflammatory. CLA also improves metabolic factors, including glucose tolerance and insulin levels, both which can reduce the risk of obesity[157] as well as promoting lean muscle mass and decreased body fat.[158]

Maximizing CLA in the Diet

One common criticism of animal studies is the frequent requirement of large doses of cancer-fighting substances required to provide a benefit. However, in these studies, a reasonable amount of CLA was consumed and often only given over a short period of time. Data from these studies reveal that only three to five weeks of consuming CLA was sufficient to fight cancer induction.[159] The question remains whether a smaller dose consumed on a daily basis for an extended time period will offer similar protection from cancer. On the typical U.S. diet, CLA consumption is around one gram per day,[160] though some data points toward Americans consuming even less at 150 mg per day.[161] Grass-fed beef generally has up to five times the amount of CLA than grain-fed cows. Regardless, recommendations to limit red meat or full-fat dairy sources will greatly reduce CLA consumption and the benefits that may accompany it.

Foods Containing CLA and Linoleic Acid
(compiled from several sources[144,145])

Food	CLA (g/kg fat)	Linoleic Acid (g/kg fat)
Dairy		
Butter	4.7	23
Milk	5.5	22
Yogurt	4.8	20
Cheese		
Cheddar	3.6	17
Cottage	4.5	22
Parmesan	3	11
Ricotta	5.6	24
Romano	2.9	11
Meat		
Ground Beef	4.3	24
Chicken	0.9	179
Lamb	5.6	58
Pork	0.6	79
Turkey	2.5	218
Veal	2.7	53
Seafood		
Salmon	0.3	102
Shrimp	0.6	16
Trout	0.5	26
Vegetable Oils		
Maize	0.2	58
Olive	0.2	79
Peanut	0.2	32
Safflower	0.7	74

When analyzing supplemental CLA there are various config-urations[162] and the data is mixed with some studies showing benefits and others as detriments.[163,164] As is often the case with nutrition, there is rarely a manufactured pill that can replace the benefit of real food and natural sources. Unfortu-nately, most of the newer studies look at supplements made from CLA derivatives.

CLA is generally only found in animal fatty tissue and in whole-fat dairy. This leaves most milk sources depleted of CLA. Skim milk is worse yet, as all valuable nutrition in the fat is removed, leaving a moderate amount of protein and a large amount of the sugar lactose. Along these lines, studies reveal that whole milk, but not skim, was associated with a decreased risk of prostate cancer in a Norwegian study.[165]

Digging deeper into the science of CLA, the amount within an animal varies widely based on the diet that the animal is fed. Over 30 years of research has shown that meat from cattle fed grass as opposed to grain has significantly more CLA, vaccenic acid, which is the precursor to CLA, and antioxidants.[166] In fact, studies show that grass-fed cows have two to five times more CLA in their meat than grain-fed counterparts.[55,166] Along these lines, the damage of grains to-ward CLA synthesis can possibly be extrapolated to humans, as we also synthesize CLA within our body.

Most recommendations have included eating three grams per day to derive the health benefits of CLA,[161] though others recommend that men should consume over six grams per day and women over four grams per day for cancer pre-vention.[160] However, to increase the amounts of CLA in the diet, harmful grains and simple sugars must be replaced with healthy fats from animal sources; the same fat that has been demonized by the medical field for several decades.

The potential for CLA to help fight cancer, while provid-ing many other health benefits, appears abundant. However, CLA is only found in fat and the animal sources that have been demonized for the past several decades.

MAXIMIZING OMEGA-3 INTAKE: TIPPING THE RATIO BACK TO HEALTH

*C*ertain fatty acids within the body cannot be produced from other fats, proteins, or carbohydrates, and thus they are an essential part of the diet and are aptly labeled as essential fats. In other words, these fats are necessary within the diet for survival. Omega-3 and omega-6 are two main essential fatty acids. Omega-3s are created from the precursor alpha-linoleic acid (ALA), and consist of eicosapentaenoic acid (EPA) and docosahexaenoic acid (DHA). Omega-6s are composed of linoleic acid as discussed above. EPA and DHA are the ingredients in fish oil capsules that are often promoted as healthy.

ALA is primarily found in the meat of free-ranging animals and wild cold-water fish. It is also found in green, leafy vegetables and even vegetable oils in small amounts. Linoleic acid is more plentiful in vegetable oils, seeds, and grains.

Similar to the discussion of the unbound carbon backbones of mono and polyunsaturated fats, the unbound carbon backbone in omega-3 and omega-6 fats is of vital importance. The '3' in omega-3 fatty acids refers to the distance of the double bond (and therefore the unbound carbon) from the end of the fatty acid. Along these lines, an omega-6 fatty acid has the bond at the sixth carbon atom from the end. This small difference in numbering results in dramatic changes within the body.

Today's modern diet has caused a shift away from the traditional and adequate proportion of omega-3 to omega-6 fatty acids. For millions of years, humans consumed nearly a 1:1 ratio of omega-6 to omega-3 fats.[42] However, in an infinitesimally small fraction of this time over the last decades and centuries, this number has increased to an astonishing 30:1 ratio[167] due to the enormous amount of omega-6s that today's modern diet contains.

The bottom arrow is pointing to the "3" in omega-3 and the top is pointing to the "6" in omega-6.

Omega-3 and Omega-6 in the Diet

A diet rich in omega-6 as opposed to omega-3 fats can lead to several health issues most likely related to an increase in inflammation. Linoleic acid, also known as omega-6, leads to inflammation and cancer, and as discussed above, is used to promote cancer in laboratory experiments. The vegetable oil and linoleic acid in these experiments acts as a vector to introduce free radicals into the body, and they result in inflammation. Population studies have shown that omega-3s appear to counteract the negative effects of omega-6s by lowering inflammatory markers like IL-6[168] and possibly even reduce the risk of certain cancers such as prostate cancer.[169,170]

DHA and EPA from omega-3s, on the other hand, contain anti-inflammatory elements that quiet inflammation and are suitably called resolvins and protectins.[171] The scientists who discovered these healing properties of DHA and EPA evidently wanted the world to acknowledge their ability to resolve and protect from inflammation.

However, both omega-3 and omega-6 fats are extremely important for many physiologic functions, including supporting the immune system, stimulating an inflammatory response, and enabling the process of blood clotting. As fats, they are both incorporated into our cell membranes as components of the cell. Yet, the body clearly has a preference and omega-6 fatty acids in the cell membranes are actually replaced by DHA and EPA from dietary omega-3s.[172] When given the choice, the body replaces inflammatory omega-6 fatty acids with inflammation-fighting omega-3s. Similar to CLA, the body appears to use the fatty acids with health benefits as the preferred cellular building blocks.

After an insult to the body, both omega fats produce inflammatory mediators; however, arachidonic acid from omega-6s is significantly more inflammatory than EPA and results in increased swelling, temperature rise, inflammation, and damage after trauma. For example, after a sprained ankle, arachidonic acid is one of the main chemicals responsible for the swelling that ensues. Interestingly, aspirin blocks this pathway and has been in use for over 2,400 years when the physician Hippocrates used it to hinder this inflammatory pathway.

Why You Should Care about Omega-6 Fats

1. Omega-6 sources are found heavily in the U.S. diet, including grains, grain-fed animals, and vegetable oils.
2. Omega-6 is composed of linoleic acid.
3. Linoleic acid is converted to arachidonic acid.
4. Arachidonic acid is a potent mediator of inflammation.
5. High omega-6 foods should be limited in an effort to keep your omega-6/omega-3 ratio under four and to reduce inflammation in your body.
6. Omega-6s increase blood vessel constriction, spasms, and blood viscosity and are prothrombotic and proaggretory, i.e. pro blood clots.
7. A high ratio of omega-6 to omega-3 is associated with an increased risk of high-grade prostate cancer.[173]

What You Need to Know about Omega-3 Fats

1. Grass-fed beef, free-roaming animals, and those fed non-grain diets have markedly higher ratios of omega-3 to omega-6.
2. Omega-3 fatty acids exhibit anti-cancer effects likely via their anti-inflammatory effects.
3. They decrease potent inflammatory factors like tumor necrosis factor (TNF) and arachidonic acid.
4. Unlike omega-6, omega-3 is antithrombotic and anti-inflammatory.
5. Omega-3s are important in the prevention and treatment of high blood pressure, diabetes, heart disease, arthritis, autoimmune disease, cancer,[167] and even macular degeneration.
6. Aiming for a 1:1 ratio of omega-6 to omega-3 may be ideal, but anything less than 4:1 is still optimal.
7. Omega-3s may fight inflammation and cancer by merely counter-acting arachidonic acid.

How to Achieve the 1:1 Ratio of Omega-6 to Omega-3

The obvious approach is to increase omega-3 consumption while decreasing omega-6. Natural sources that are high in omega-3 include grass-fed beef, vegetables, and wild-caught fish. Similar to CLA, grass-fed beef has four-times the omega-3s than confined and grain-fed cattle. Cream and cheese from these ruminants have more omega-3s as well.[174] The same goes for fish[175] and eggs;[176] wild salmon contains ample amounts of omega-3s while farmed salmon contains a large amount of inflammatory omega-6s.

Much of the world's farmed fish supply comes from Southeast Asia allowing consumers to easily identify it from the packaging. Unlike farm-raised salmon, DHA, the omega-3 that our brain is made of, is increased in the cell membranes of cold-water fish to keep them warm. If salmon are raised in warm water conditions, such as the farms of Southeast Asia, they will not build up DHA omega-3, significantly decreasing their nutritional value.

Interestingly, cultured vegetables are no different and contain significantly less omega-3s than their wild counterparts.[167] Just as omega-3 is a fat, good food sources of omega-3 must also contain fat; this provides one of the many instances where the avoidance of fat may lead to poorer health.

In conclusion, both omega-3 and omega-6 fatty acids are a necessary component of the diet providing many physiologic benefits. Even the increases in inflammation that occur from omega-6s are necessary to fight infection and other insults to the body. Unfortunately, modern foods and techniques of industrially raising animals has brought upon an abundance of omega-6s. Yet, attempts can be made to correct this balance by avoiding vegetable oils, grains, and other foods high in omega-6s, and in turn, this out-of-balance ratio may once again approach what was initially intended for the human body.

Omega-3 and Cancer

1. A recent mouse study at Wake Forest University revealed that DHA blocked survival pathways in breast cancer cells causing these cancer cells to undergo apoptosis, a form of cell death.[177]
2. Omega-3s have been shown to decrease the incidence and enhance the treatment of colon cancer.[178]
3. Omega-3s stop prostate cancer progression by blocking proliferation pathways like mTOR, whereas omega-6 arachidonic acid actually promotes tumor progression.[179]
4. High levels of omega-3 fatty acids in actual breast tissue obtained through biopsy or lumpectomy were associated with a lower risk of breast cancer, and the amount of DHA in the breasts of cancer patients correlated with their response to chemotherapy.[180]

10

FIGHTING CANCER BY COOKING WITH SATURATED FAT

"Fat gives things flavor."
–Julia Childs, famous chef and author

While it is apparent that the recommendation to avoid saturated fats and replace them with polyunsaturated vegetable oils is based on minimal research, the health issues become more apparent when cooking with these oils. The health aspects of cooking oils are closely associated with the structure of the oil, the smoke point, and of course, how the oil is made. Systematically assessing each of these aspects provides insight into which fats and oils may be preferable in regards to heath.

Smoke Point

Oils are created out of glycerol and fatty acids, and when exposed to heat they break down into these two components. This point is called the smoke point, or the temperature at which the oil starts to burn and smoke. Once this occurs, the oil essentially becomes rancid and free radicals and oxidation start forming within. Glycerol in the oil is converted to acrolein, a chemical that is found in cigarette smoke and is considered to be one of the most prominent cancer-causing agents from smoking.[181] It damages DNA and renders cells unable to fix the damage, which can lead to cancer. Studies have shown that acrolein can cause both lung and bladder cancer.[182]

In fact, fumes from peanut oil[183] and canola oil,[184] two common vegetable oils used to replace saturated fats for "health benefit," have been shown to cause lung cancer when inhaled. Along these lines, there has been an increase of prevalence in young Asian women diagnosed with lung cancer even when they have no history of smoking. Newer studies are revealing data that implicates inhaled vegetable oil fumes during cooking as a cause of lung damage and cancer.[185,186] Acrolein also activates the endothelial growth factor receptor (EGFR),[187] a receptor that, when mutated, leads to lung cancer. This gene is also frequently amplified in young Asian women with lung cancer and no history of smoking.

As discussed previously, heating oil to its smoke point also oxidizes the fatty acids, resulting in the accumulation of free radicals and potentially destroying any antioxidant benefits. In conclusion, heating oil above its smoke point releases toxic chemicals, damages the oil, and introduces free radicals that are harmful to your body.

Smoke Points of Oils

225° F
Canola Oil, Unref.
Flaxseed Oil, Unref.
Safflower Oil, Unref.
Sunflower Oil, Unref.

320° F
Olive Oil, Unref.
Peanut Oil, Unref.
Safflower Oil, Semi-Ref.
Soybean Oil, Unref.
Walnut Oil, Unref.

325° F
Hemp Seed Oil

330° F
Butter

350° F
Canola Oil, Semi-Ref.
Coconut Oil
Sesame Oil, Unref.
Soybean Oil, Semi-Ref.
Corn Oil, Unref.
Vegetable Shortening

375° F
Olive Oil, Extra Virgin
Canola Oil, Ref.

400° F
Walnut Oil, Semi-Refined
Avocado Oil

410° F
Macadamia Oil
Cottonseed Oil

420° F
Olive Oil, Virgin
Almond Oil
Hazelnut Oil
Grapeseed Oil

440° F
Corn Oil, Ref.

450° F
Peanut Oil, Ref.
Safflower Oil, Ref.
Sesame Oil, Semi-Ref.
Soybean Oil, Ref.
Sunflower Oil, Semi-Ref.

455° F
Palm Oil

485° F
Ghee (Clarified Butter)

Legend: *Smoke Points of Oils: the temperature at which the oil becomes damaged and starts to smoke. These values can vary based on processing and oil composition, but serve to give a general idea of the smoke points. (Ref.- refined, Unref.- unrefined)*

Polyunsaturated Fats

One method to combat the damage that occurs from heating oil is to cook with more stable oils. As discussed above, saturated fat is more stable than unsaturated fat, which leaves it solid at room temperature. The difference between saturated and unsaturated fat is that the saturated fat is *saturated* with hydrogen atoms bound to the carbon backbone while unsaturated fats have less hydrogen atoms attached leaving many unbound carbon atoms on its backbone. These bound hydrogen atoms keep saturated fats stable, but also help protect it against oxidation and the binding of free radicals during cooking.

Since polyunsaturated fats are less stable, they tend to break down into oxidized products during storage and when exposed to light, oxygen, and even non-cooking temperatures. Placing these oils in high heat only compounds these issues. While Canola and peanut oil have been recommended as healthy cooking oils by mainstream health sources since they are unsaturated, it becomes obvious as to why the exact opposite may be true.

Shelf Life of Oils

Oil	Shelf Life (months)
Coconut	12
Palm	12
Avocado	12
Canola	12
Corn	9-12
Olive	6-12
Macadamia	6-12
Almond	6-12
Safflower	6
Soybean	6
Peanut	6
Grape Seed	3-6
Sunflower	3
Walnut	2-4
Sesame	2-4

Legend: *Shelf Life of Oils: similar to the smoke point, when these oils reach their shelf life, they become damaged and begin to oxidize. The healthiest cooking oils are bolded.*

There are three main benefits of cooking with more structurally sound saturated and monounsaturated fats versus polyunsaturated fats and vegetable oils:

1. Less heat-induced degradation during cooking
2. Less degradation during storage and longer shelf life
3. Less or no defenseless areas where free radicals can attack and bind

When these weak fats become damaged, degraded, and bound with free radicals, they can potentially lead to atherosclerosis, inflammatory joint disease, rheumatoid arthritis, damage to the GI tract, and mutagenicity and genotoxicity, which can lead to birth defects and cancer.[188] Chronic ingestion of oxidized unsaturated lipids in oil increases atherosclerosis and cancer incidence in animals. When ingested, these oxidized lipids have also been shown to damage liver cells and lymphocytes, the same cells that fight infection and cancer.[189]

Oxidized cholesterol also collects on artery walls and is attacked by macrophages to form atherosclerotic plaques, or in other words, heart disease. Studies have even shown that oxidized lipids are absorbed and directly sent into the bloodstream where they can wreak havoc on the walls of arteries and organs.[190]

Saturated Fats: Are They Responsible for Clogged Arteries?

Interestingly, it is quite possible that while fats alone may not be the main culprits behind atherosclerosis, oxidized unsaturated fats and their oxidized constituents may be a contributor through similar mechanisms that cause inflammation and cancer (as discussed above). In fact, palm oil, which contains almost fifty percent saturated fat, has been shown to reduce the risk of atherosclerosis, arterial clots, and blood pressure, and also inhibit platelet aggregation and cholesterol biosynthesis.[191]

However, it also contains a significant amount of polyunsaturated fats, and when oxidized by high heat and repetitive usage, it has been shown to result in an unhealthy plasma lipid profile, as well as damage to the kidneys, lungs, liver, and heart.[192] Polyunsaturated fats from vegetable oils have also been shown to promote cancer over saturated fats or polyunsaturated fish fat sources.[138] A randomized trial that replaced saturated fats with unsaturated fats revealed a large increase in lung cancer rates at the conclusion of the study.[139]

The potential for oxidation does not only happen on the shelf or when cooking at high heat. The warm and acidic environment of the stomach has also been shown to cause damage and oxidation to unstable fats after consumption,[193] as does heating them in the microwave.[194] However, even in the microwave, higher percentages of saturated fat in the lipid results in less oxidation, while the opposite occurs with polyunsaturated fats.

If inflammation is in fact the main culprit for the accumulation of plaques within the arteries, perhaps removing the source that introduces this inflammation via oxidation will be most beneficial. In fact, in a study assessing the dietary intake of individuals and the amount of buildup within their aortas on biopsy found that it was directly proportional to the amount of polyunsaturated fats within their diet.[195]

In conclusion, the stability of oil, often meaning the oil with the least amount of polyunsaturated fat, will be the most stable and defend against oxidation and free radical formation in the stomach, on the shelf, in the frying pan, and likely in the arteries.

Stability of Cooking Oils and Fats

Oil/Fat	Saturated	MUFA	PUFA
Macadamia	16%	83%	1%
Coconut	92%	6%	2%
Lard	41%	47%	2%
Ghee	65%	32%	3%
Butter	66%	30%	4%
Sunflower	9%	82%	9%
Palm	51%	39%	10%
Olive	14%	73%	11%
Avocado	12%	74%	14%
Mustard	13%	60%	21%
Almond	8%	66%	26%
Canola	6%	62%	32%
Rice Bran	20%	47%	33%
Peanut	18%	49%	33%
Sesame	14%	43%	43%
Cottonseed	24%	26%	50%
Soybean	15%	24%	61%

Legend: Structural Backbone of Oils: they are listed in order of polyunsaturated fat (PUFA) percentage. The less the polyunsaturated fat component, the more stable they are for cooking. The healthiest cooking oils are bolded. (MUFA–monounsaturated fat)

Artificially Hydrogenated Trans-Fats

While the process of turning a vegetable or plant-based fare into oil requires an intricate process, the creation of trans-fats takes this process one step further to artificially solidify them. This same process keeps artificial peanut butter creamy, while natural peanut butter separates over time leaving a liquid floating at the top of the jar. The process of hydrogenation ensures that the peanut oil stays solid by blasting the polyunsaturated oil with hydrogens to artificially "saturate" the fat. This process of solidification makes these products difficult to break down in the jar and within the body after they are digested.

Similar to omega-6 and omega-3 fatty acids, trans-fats are incorporated into the body's cell walls. The less stable structure of the omega fatty acids is desired as the fluidity can allow nutrients to pass through the cell wall and into the cell, but trans-fats, on the other hand, inhibit the ability of the cell walls to adequately let nutrients pass. They also disrupt cellular receptors that are located along the cell wall, such as the insulin receptor,[196] and may lead to cardiovascular disease and heart attacks.[197]

A polyunsaturated fat is bombarded with hydrogen molecules at the arrows:

This results in an artificially created saturated fat:

Revisiting the Omega 3:6 Ratio

As discussed previously, our natural dietary ratio of 1:1 to 4:1 of omega-6 to omega-3 fatty acids has ballooned to over 30:1 with the advent of grains, grain-fed animals, and vegetable oils. As increased omega-6 consumption can lead to inflammation, circulatory issues, and even cancer, fat sources or oils with the highest amounts of omega-3s and the fewest omega-6s, are likely optimal in cooking oils as well. Linoleic acid, the prime source of omega-6 in vegetable oils, seeds, and grains should be avoided. For instance, sources like linoleic sunflower oil provide 65.7 grams omega-6 per 100 gram serving with no omega-3. Consuming enough omega-3s to balance this ratio would be difficult, if not impossible.

Adding It All Up

Reviewing all of the above properties of fats and cooking oil, several sources consistently have high smoke points, few polyunsaturated fats, low omega-6 fatty acid content, and are not processed vegetable oils. These are the same food sources that have been demonized for several decades. It is also apparent that several of these are the sources that were replaced by the now outlawed trans-fats. The most common oils that have these properties, in no specific order are:

1. Macadamia nut oil
2. Avocado oil
3. Grass-fed butter
4. Ghee (clarified grass-fed butter)
5. Palm oil
6. Coconut oil
7. Olive oil (often avoided for high heat cooking due to smoke point)
8. Lard/tallow

Omega-3 Fatty Acid Component

Oil/Fat	Omega-3	Omega-6
Macadamia Oil	0.2	1.3
Coconut Oil	0	1.8
Cocoa Butter	0.1	2.8
Sunflower Oil	0.2	3.6
Palm Oil	0.2	9.1
Olive Oil	0.8	9.8
Hazelnut Oil	0	10.1
Avocado Oil	1	12.5
Flaxseed Oil	53.3	12.7
Safflower Oil	0	14.4
Almond Oil	0	17.4
Canola Oil	9.1	18.7
Peanut Oil	0	31.7
Rice Bran Oil	1.6	33.4
Sesame Oil	0.3	41.3
Soybean Oil	6.8	50.4
Cottonseed Oil	0.2	51.5

Legend: *Omega-3 and Omega-6 Components of Fats: fats with more omega-3s (listed in grams) and less omega-6s (listed in grams) are generally the healthiest. The healthiest fats are bolded.*

PART THREE

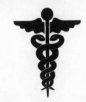

GUIDING YOUR LIFESTYLE

"The doctor of the future will give no medicines, but will interest his patients in the care of the human frame, in diet, and in the causes and prevention of disease."
–Thomas Edison

THE VITAMIN TAKEOVER

"To all my little Hulkamaniacs, say your prayers, take your vitamins and you will never go wrong."
    –Hulk Hogan,
        professional wrestler, actor, and television personality

After fat was thoroughly chastised for several decades, the amount of fatty food in the diet was reduced, and many of these left-out foods included nutrient-dense animal products. As a result, the amount of vitamins within the diet began to fall and had to be replenished in another way. Adding to the issue, processed grains have little digestible nutritional value and must be enriched with factory-produced vitamins and nutrients.

The foods that historically supplied humans with large amounts of vitamins and nutrients were castigated and removed based on little data, and thus the vitamin movement was born. The American people no longer needed to get their nutrients from food, as they could simply supply their bodies with the necessary vitamins, nutrients, and minerals in a convenient pill. The mainstream health leaders welcomed the vitamin movement with open arms. While physicians were slow to jump aboard, the vitamin movement became another misguided health movement.

The vitamin industry is an enormous business with $23 billion in domestic sales annually. Malls traditionally contained one General Nutrition Center (GNC), but now frequently contain a GNC, Vitamin Shoppe, and Vitamin World, along with drug stores like Walgreens and Rite Aid. Congruently, the food court contains vitamin-sparse refined foods as well. However, recent data reveals vitamins to be inferior to food itself, and these simple, convenient pills may prove less than adequate.

Take, for instance, Dr. Terry Wahls who developed the incurable disease, multiple sclerosis, also known as MS. In MS, the body begins to attack itself for unknown reasons. This attack takes place in the white matter of the brain, and its victims are left with a plethora of symptoms, including speech dysfunction and decreased motor function, often leading to the inability to walk. Dr. Wahls, once a national Tae Kwon Do champion, found herself confined to a wheelchair.

Modern treatments consisting of thousands of dollars of expensive drugs were not working as her disease continued to progress.[198] She decided to take her heath into her own hands and spent countless hours researching the causes of MS. She found that feeding her mitochondria, the important organelle known as the powerhouse of our cells, might be the key to the cure. To go along with her discovery, she took dozens of vitamins and supplements that would aid her mitochondria in growth, repair, and function. The vitamins worked to stop her disease from progressing, which was a step in the right direction from her expensive medications but still not a cure.

In another effort to achieve remission with her disease, she decided to replace her modern, nutrient-sparse diet that consisted of foods like wheat with foods rich in vitamins and nutrients that are necessary for optimal mitochondrial function, like leafy green vegetables. Some of the most nutrient-dense foods she included were not only leafy green vegetables, but also foods like organ meats and animal products that were high in saturated fat. Such a diet stood counter to what was recommended and proposed to her as healthy for several decades. As she consumed this diet, one that resembled that of her ancestors, she went from being bed-ridden to returning to her life as a physician and even riding a bike to work.[199] Her cure of an incurable disease with diet alone has inspired her to tell the story of her journey through a TED Talk, and she has incorporated her "treatment" into clinical trials.

Returning to modern foods, many components of a "healthy" diet include bread and grains, which have to be fortified with synthesized vitamins and nutrients to account for their deficits. The diet of modern-day hunter-gatherers, whose diets may more closely mimic that of our ancestors, such as those of the Innuit and Maasai tribes, provide over double and even up to 10 times the recommended daily allowance of vitamins and nutrients.[200]

The Inuit, considered the Eskimos of the North, and Maasai, the Kenyan tribesmen, are a modern example of a group of people who continue to eat an ancient diet. Their diets consist of mostly saturated fat and are heavy with animal products, including the fatty portions and organ meat, and these sources of food are extremely nutrient-dense and are higher in vitamins, minerals, antioxidants, phytochemicals, protein, fiber, and omega-3 fatty acids.[201] This includes the Inuit Eskimos in the far north who drink no milk nor take calcium pills. The history of humans provides many clues to what a diet for optimal health should be, and in Dr. Wahls' case, it allowed her to provide the first ever cure for multiple sclerosis.

Vitamins and Nutrients in Food versus Pills

There are clearly instances where supplementation provides benefits, as certain medical conditions can lead to roadblocks in normal eating. For instance, certain cancer patients are unable to consume a normal diet due to difficulty swallowing or digestion issues. However, rarely should the backbone of a healthy diet require supplementation. Often these supplements include processed substances and vegetable oils, which are used as fillers, adding to the potential issues as previously discussed.

Under the guidance of the food pyramid and mainstream dietary recommendations, a typical western diet has resulted in over half of the U.S. population failing to meet the recommended dietary allowance (RDA) for vitamin A, vitamin B-6, magnesium, calcium, and zinc,[202] and one-third of the population is under the RDA for folate. This diet, which provides a trifling amount of vitamins and minerals,[203] provides a fraction of a diet based upon animal foods and plants.

Several studies reveal the result of supplementing this nutrient-poor diet with vitamins. In fact, studies with antioxidants provide a bird's eye view of the consequence of supplementing with vitamins rather than getting them naturally from our food sources.

As free radical bombardment upon the body results in significant inflammation and other health issues, antioxidants became an easy target for studies assessing supplementation. This inflammation can be minimized and combated through diet, exercise, and lifestyle. Researchers turned to vitamins and pills instead, but similar to Dr. Wahls' experience, the results revealed the pitfalls of avoiding a nutrient-dense diet and instead relying on the convenience of powders and pills.

One of the first major studies undertaken was the MRD/ BHF Heart Protection Study, where half of adults with cardiovascular disease or diabetes were given vitamin E, vitamin C, and beta carotene, while the other half were given a placebo.[204] Results revealed no significant reduction in mortality from vascular disease or cancer. Similar studies in women given these vitamins[205] and others where they were given B vitamins also showed no benefit.[206,207] Epidemiologic data reveals that obtaining vitamin C through fruits and leafy green vegetables is correlated with a decreased risk of heart disease.[208] However, in Italy the GISSI-Prevenzione Trial supplied patients with omega-3s and vitamin E and found that omega-3s were beneficial, but the antioxidant vitamin E was not.[209] Fish oil may be somewhat of an extenuating circumstance as they are made directly from the source of fish, though data is unclear.

Further studies started to reveal a *detriment* with the addition of vitamins and antioxidants. One of the most famous of these studies was the SELECT Trial where researchers supplemented men with selenium and vitamin E to help reduce the risk of prostate cancer.[210] They unexpectedly found that not only was there no benefit for these men, but vitamin E supplementation trended towards an *increase* in prostate cancer. More worrisome, the Norwegian Vitamin Trial and Western Norway B Vitamin Intervention Trial A supplemented women with heart disease with folic acid and vitamin B12 and found that it *increased* the risk of cancer and death.[211] Such results should have rocked the vitamin industry, yet, these trials remain relatively unknown by the mainstream media.

More worrisome is the fact that many foods now have vitamins added into them to attempt to offset their poor nutrient density. Grains, for example, are generally poor sources of digestible nutrients and they are often supplemented with vitamins. Grains in the U.S. are fortified with folic acid, further adding to their potential health detriments based on results from the study above. Folic acid is dissimilar to naturally occurring folate, and data has been accumulating that excess folic acid may lead to increased cancer risk. Folic acid supplementation may also promote cancer growth, cardiovascular disease, and inhibit immune function.[212] Along these lines, when scientists attempted to supplement with CLA in pill form, the benefits did not translate and similar health detriments occurred.

While information on vitamins is generally negative or neutral, vitamin D is one of the few that reveals conclusive positive data. A major analysis of 50 randomized trials with over 94,000 participants, mostly elderly women, took place assessing vitamin D supplementation.[213] The results showed that supplementation with Vitamin D3 reduced mortality, while vitamin D2 did not. Vitamin D is produced within the skin when exposed to the sun, and it may actually provide a benefit in pill form due to the fact that throughout certain times of the year or due to work, many are unable to get adequate sun exposure.

Interestingly, these studies may reveal why many vitamin studies may yield negative results. Vitamin D2 is a synthesized version of vitamin D, derived from a cell membrane produced by fungi and plankton when they are exposed to UV light. Vitamin D3 is the naturally occurring form within the body and it has greater bioefficacy than D2.[214] In conclusion, nutrient sources within actual food or closest to natural sources are often the healthiest.

Nutrient-Dense Foods, the Natural Source of Vitamins

The most nutrient-dense foods have often received the most criticism by the medical field, as they often have the largest amounts of fat and calories. For instance, beef provides significant amounts of iron, zinc, selenium, folic acid, and vitamins

A, B6, B12, D, and, E.[215] Beef, once again, is in stark contrast to foods like wheat, which are so severely nutrient-deficient, they must have synthesized vitamins added to enrich them, even though these vitamins have been shown to increase the risk of cancer and death.

Returning to the history of humans, the diet mostly consisted of wild plants, animals, and fish for millions of years, all naturally high sources of vitamins and nutrients. Our bodies have adjusted to consume these same foods, as represented by these studies, not pills. Along these lines, several studies have compared those who eat a modern day version of this same animal-based and nutrient-dense diet with that of vegetarians. The Lugalawa study in Tanzania[216] and data from the west coast Eskimos in Greenland[217] have revealed that the nutrient-dense animal-consumers have lower blood pressure, superior cholesterol levels, and lower triglycerides than vegetarians.

Common Nutrient-Dense Foods

Kale:
1. 206% daily value (DV) vitamin A
2. 134% DV vitamin C
3. 684% DV vitamin K
4. 26% DV manganese
5. 90.5 mg calcium
6. 22.8 mg magnesium
7. 19.4 mcg folate
8. 299 mg potassium

Red Meat:
1. 86% DV of niacin
2. 78% DV vitamin B6
3. 45% DV vitamin B12
4. 97% DV selenium
5. 67% DV zinc
6. 52% DV phosphorous
7. 22% iron

Eggs:
1. 21% DV vitamin D
2. 68% DV riboflavin
3. 29% DV folate
4. 46% phosphorous
5. 52% vitamin B12
6. 35% DV pantothenic acid
7. 110% selenium

Wild and Unfarmed Salmon:
1. 4 g omega 3 fatty acids
2. 78% DV niacin
3. 105% DV vitamin B12
4. 103% selenium
5. 44% riboflavin
6. 30% thiamin

12

CALCIUM: PROTECTING BONES OR DAMAGING THE HEART?

"A vigorous five-mile walk will do more good for an unhappy but otherwise healthy adult than all the medicine and psychology in the world."
—Paul Dudley White, M.D., prominent cardiologist

*T*he abandonment of nutrient-dense foods within the diet brought about the reliance on vitamins. With this, the food pyramid recommended calcium-rich dairy, often in the form of low-fat or skim milk, creating another major misguided health movement of the 20th century. Calcium was one of the most common vitamins recommended due to its potential bone health benefit. This is a paramount example of medicine choosing a vitamin over the superior health benefits derived from diet and exercise.

The dietary recommendation to consume more milk and dairy parallels the push for more calcium. The fact that humans have historically subsided on a diet much lower in calcium than is currently recommended is often ignored. Also forgotten, the largest nutrient provided in milk, and especially skim milk, is the sugar lactose. Worse off, many of the benefits of dairy are found in its fat content, which is removed with commonly endorsed low-fat milk.

A closer look at the calcium phenomenon uncovers that many factors affect calcium levels and bone health, not just the amount of calcium consumed. Increasing blood calcium levels and incorporating calcium from the blood and into the bones are entirely different entities. This process involves several steps, including calcium consumption to increase the blood serum levels, extracting the calcium from the blood and into the bones to aid in bone formation, and limiting the loss of calcium from the body during excretion. The body constantly orchestrates an intricate interplay between all of these factors while implementing hormonal manipulation to aid in this coordination.

A polarized view of calcium and bone health as simply the factor of input is not only incorrect but dangerous. Hospitalizations from levels of calcium that are dangerously high continue to increase due to the markedly increased rate of over-the-counter calcium supplement use.[218] Yet, people are continually told to take more calcium pills and drink more milk, a food that is relatively new in the history of humans.

At the end of the day, Americans consume the largest amount of calcium-rich foods like dairy along with a large amount of calcium supplementation, yet they have some of the highest rates of osteoporosis. These issues are not singular to the United States. In Greece, the rate of hip fractures has steadily climbed[219] while the consumption of milk has skyrocketed. Once again, calcium intake is only one of several factors affecting bone health, and dwelling on this aspect alone will neglect the other important components.

Calcium Absorption

The first step in increasing available calcium is consumption, and the next step is actually absorbing it within the gastrointestinal tract. Several factors in the diet may limit the absorption of calcium. Phytic acid, found in significant amounts in grains, binds to calcium and greatly decreases the gut's ability to absorb it.[220,221] The absorption of calcium within the gut also relies on a healthy intestinal tract. Gluten and lectin, also from grains and legumes (beans and peanuts), damage the lining of the intestines resulting in significant inflammation further impairing intake.

Studies also reveal that higher levels of serum vitamin D lead to drastically increased amounts of calcium absorption.[222] In those with inflammatory bowel disease, increases in inflammation are associated with lower vitamin D levels.[223] Studies also reveal that physicians frequently overlook vitamin D depletion as the cause of osteoporosis,[224] and this is likely due to the fact that the emphasis is more often placed on calcium alone. In regards to calcium absorption, raising levels through increases in dietary calcium become futile in the face of a diet high in grains or with low levels of vitamin D.

Bone Construction

Just as the process of bringing calcium into the body relies on more factors than just consumption, converting this calcium into healthy bone is just as intricate. Bone mineralization relies on multiple vitamins and nutrients and is significantly dependent on vitamin D and vitamin K2 intake.[99] Vitamin K is found in large amounts in green, leafy vegetables, such as broccoli and spinach,[225] and vitamin K2 is found in fatty sources, like organ meats, fatty dairy such as cheese and butter, egg yolks, and ground beef. Calcium is often found in green, leafy vegetables like kale, and is significantly more absorbable than dairy calcium. These green vegetables provide a highly absorbable form of calcium and a generous amount of vitamin K, which helps to further absorb subsequent calcium. Low-fat dairy, however, remains a poor source of vitamin K and to add insult to injury, contains a much less absorbable source of calcium.[226]

Protein also has a stimulatory effect on the synthesis of bones. Studies have shown that supplementing elderly patients and postmenopausal women with protein increases bone density, reduces bone loss on x-ray, and improves clinical symptoms in patients with recent hip fractures.[227-229] Increased protein consumption results in several anabolic (growth) processes, including bone formation, and is not just limited to muscle growth. It appears that when vitamin D and K are present with protein, calcium is pulled from the blood to stimulate bone formation.

Physical Activity and Bone Construction

Increased physical activity[99] and more specifically lifting heavy weights and resistance training increases bone mineralization. In fact, exercising the muscles via resistance or weight-bearing exercise can increase bone mineral content and density by up to five percent a year.[230] Just as weight training stresses muscles, leading to damage repair and bigger and stronger muscle fibers, bone follows a similar pattern. Sprinting causes a similar stress on the shin and leg bones leading to increased strength.

When scientists observed bone scans of the tibias in the lower legs of long-distance runners, sprinters, and walkers, sprinters appear to have the healthiest bone structure. The acute impact from sprinting appears to provide enough stress to stimulate bone construction.[231] Regardless of the exact method of resistance, the bony skeleton clearly requires the encounter of periodic heavy resistance as the body responds with an increase in bone density and strength as it prepares our bones for the next physical challenge. Higher intensity exercise appears to provide the largest benefit.[232]

Calcium Secretion

Returning to vitamin D, not only does it help the body absorb more calcium, but it also activates the kidney to reabsorb calcium. This process stops it from being secreted in the urine. In fact, studies show vitamin D levels to be the dominant predictor of bone density and not calcium.[233] This may once again point to the history of human beings, as they frequently encountered the sun's rays, which stimulate vitamin D, while the traditional human diet had very few sources of calcium.

Several other factors act on the kidney to affect calcium loss in the urine. Insulin, the hormone secreted after carbohydrate consumption to lower the ensuing rise in blood sugar, negatively affects calcium secretion as well. Insulin binds to receptors on the kidneys, activates them, and signals to the kidney to release calcium in the urine, in turn, increasing calcium loss.[234] Interestingly, a diet high in carbohydrates and similar to that advocated by mainstream medicine and the food pyramid leads to massive surges of insulin and increased calcium loss in the kidneys.[235] While the numbers are not exact, it becomes clear that as one lowers the amount of carbohydrates in the diet, thus stimulating less insulin, the requirement of calcium will lessen as well.

Unfortunately, as is often the case in the modern era, the body's natural physiologic mechanisms for increasing and maintaining bone strength were largely ignored. Physicians and patients turned to dairy, including skim milk, which is mostly composed of the insulin-raising sugar lactose. Even more misguided was the constant recommendation for calcium supplementation. Not only does calcium supplementation in isolation ignore nearly all of the physiologic methods within the body to strengthen the bones, but it may be outright dangerous; recent data has revealed this danger. When a pathologist removes the contents of a blocked coronary artery after a heart attack, a significant portion of the blockage is actually calcium. Common sense would lead to the conclusion that isolated supplementation of calcium without the ability to pull it from the circulation and into the bone could lead to accumulation within the blood and therefore arteries.

Recent studies have revealed the dangers of calcium supplementation. This data has shown that calcium supplementation in healthy older women is associated with a higher rate of heart attacks.[236] A study of nearly 400,000 individuals has revealed an increase in cardiovascular death in men who took calcium supplements.[237] A large European study confirmed these results, revealing an increased risk of heart attack with calcium pills but not necessarily with dietary calcium.[238] Interestingly, data reveal that elevated blood calcium levels in women are associated with death from heart disease,[239] once again pointing to the risk from elevated calcium in the blood that is not pulled into the bone.

Data in mice further illustrates this point. It reveals that supplementation with vitamin K reduces calcium plaques in the arteries, pulling the excess calcium from the blood and placing it in the bones, where it belongs.[240] Cholesterol, a vital substance for life, has been chastised for being found in arterial blockages, while calcium, also found in these blockages, has been the most common supplement recommended in doctors' offices across the U.S. As one would expect, the data is accumulating that this recommendation has had ominous health consequences.

Other efforts have included estrogen replacement, as this female hormone appears to aid in bone synthesis, but decreases with menopause.[241] Unfortunately, these efforts resulted in an increased risk of several cancers, including endometrial[242] and breast cancer;[243] both topics received large media coverage. As a result, this treatment is appropriately avoided in most cases.

Instead, physicians often turn to another medication, called Reclast, which has been shown to reduce the occurrence of hip fracture from 2.5 to 1.4% and vertebral fractures from 10.9 to 3.3% at the expense of an increased risk of atrial fibrillation, known as an irregular heartbeat,[244] potentially from resulting mineral deficiencies as it can cause lower levels of calcium and magnesium in the blood than the body requires. Joint pain can occur in nearly a fourth of patients, along with muscle pain, fever, headaches and high blood pressure, all factors that may decrease a person's ability to exercise, which stimulates bone strength and an array of other health benefits. Such effects would clearly have detrimental effects on many other aspects of health, including weight gain and high blood pressure as this drug may lead to a sedentary lifestyle.

Another drug frequently recommended is Fosamax, which actually works similarly to exercise and decreases bone breakdown and favors bone formation.[245] A main difference between the two is that exercise also contributes many other health benefits like stress relief, increased insulin sensitivity, and weight loss. Fosamax, on the other hand, often causes muscle and bone pain and even osteonecrosis, which paradoxically is when bone dies and undergoes a process called necrosis.

Milk and calcium supplements are not only unnecessary for proper bone health, but they are actually mediocre sources. The history of humans reveals that a diet absent of calcium supplements and even milk may be optimal for bone health. This diet, with lower amounts of carbohydrates and insulin and higher amounts of fat sources containing vitamins D and

K2, coupled with weight-bearing exercise is the key to bone health and avoiding osteoporosis. Isolated supplementation is not only ineffective but may be hazardous to our heath.

What You Need to Know about Calcium:

1. Calcium levels and bone health are multifactorial and calcium intake is only one aspect of bone health.
2. Calcium from dairy is less absorbable than calcium from some vegetables.
3. Avoiding foods that result in decreased calcium absorption and increased excretion of calcium may be a better strategy than over-consuming calcium.
4. Sun exposure significantly increases the natural production of vitamin D.
5. Lifting weights and sprinting stimulates bone mineralization and decreases bone breakdown.
6. Highly absorbable sources of calcium include green leafy vegetables like broccoli, while milk is a poorly absorbable source, and it has a large amount of insulin-stimulating sugar per serving.
7. Avoiding large amounts of carbohydrates in the diet may help to decrease insulin release and calcium loss in the kidneys.

THE MARATHON
MOVEMENT

"If you feel bad at 10 miles, you're in trouble. If you feel bad at 20 miles, you're normal. If you don't feel bad at 26 miles, you're abnormal."
—Rob de Castella, 1983 World Marathon
Championship winner

490 BC*.* The time of year was August, and Greece and Persia were battling in Marathon. Greece emerged victorious, and Pheidippides, a proud citizen of Greece, took it upon himself to sprint the nearly 22-mile distance from Marathon to Athens to spread the news.

Upon entering the assembly, excited and shouting, "We have won," he fell over dead. And so was the story of the first marathon. Most would think that people clearly realized that exerting the body to such extremes and running extended distances could never be healthy, since Pheidippides was a young, healthy, trained soldier and yet it killed him. As a result, one would also surmise that marathon running, jogging, and endurance training would be abandoned as the health risks of continuous exercise were known by all. Yet, each year on the third Monday of April, we actually commemorate Pheidippides and his selfless act of revealing the dangers of long-distance running and endurance training by holding a marathon in Boston. Since then, we have come to realize the benefits of different forms of exercise like sprinting, walking frequently, and lifting heavy objects.

Unfortunately, while many have begun to realize the benefits of sprinting, walking, and resistance training, the lessons learned from Pheidippides have been minimal at best. As is often the case with mankind, we chose to ignore our history and important life lessons. The third Monday of April each year is celebrated as Patriots' Day, also known as the day of the annual Boston Marathon. Over the last 30 years, physicians, trainers, and many more have prescribed jogging and endurance exercise as the cure-all for diabetes, hypertension, obesity, and heart disease, among others. Weight training was left to the bodybuilders, like Lou Ferrigno, and sprinting was left to the Olympians like Michael Johnson. Jogging and endurance training were prescribed as the pathway to health for everyone else. Those who competed in marathons and triathlons were considered the paragons of health.

In the late 1970s, around the same time our government released the "Dietary Guidelines for Americans," and obesity rates began to rise dramatically, recommendations for jogging and endurance training started accumulating and took off over the next several decades. The most common product of the marathon and jogging movement is middle-aged males frequently seen jogging through the neighborhood, accumulating dozens of miles per week for decades.

These recommendations were based on several studies revealing that, in essence, the more activity one engaged in, the less chance he or she had of dying from heart disease[246] or cancer,[247] and the more intense the exercise, the better.[248] Specifically, many studies had revealed exercise capacity to be the major predictor of a reduction in mortality from exercise.[249,250] In the typical bigger, stronger, faster American approach, if increased exercise capacity on a treadmill revealed benefits in health, then excessive amounts of jogging and endurance training must be even more beneficial. While such a mentality may have brought Americans amazing technological creations from producing some of the world's best cars at the turn of the century and revolutionizing industry through the mass production of steel, this mentality rarely leads to improvements in health.

Much like the anti-fat campaign, such misguided recommendations were an attempt to promote health but missed the mark. These recommendations never approached the question as to whether the human body was ever equipped to handle such constant wear and tear throughout its history and whether the joints, heart, and bones were meant to withstand such excessive stress and pounding. It was also difficult to ascertain whether these studies simply supported the notion that active individuals were simply healthier than those who followed a sedentary lifestyle.

How Did Man Exercise over the past Million Years?

The simple answer: he did not. For millions of years humans have walked miles per day in search of food and water, sprinted in short bursts from predators and after prey, and lifted heavy objects while performing manual labor and hunting. Even gathering food required intense climbing, bending, squatting, digging, and lifting.[251] This likely did not include extensive periods of continuous running like jogging, not to mention marathons. Man did not engage in endurance training, especially not under the guise of health.

Circumstances may have led to exceptions of course, but it seems as most of the exercise man encountered during his upright evolution involved periods of high intensity activity in short spurts intermixed with lifting of heavy weights and long periods of walking[251] – both the antithesis of endurance training and jogging. In this regard, exercise was by accident. Unfortunately, our society seems to have reached a paradox: physical activity is decreasing in many, even children;[252] however, jogging, an exercise activity previously unseen in our society, has increased exponentially in the past several decades.[253]

The modern-day hunter-gatherers also give a glimpse into past-time activities, as the Ache in eastern Paraguay have been known to walk extremely long distances intermixed with 20-30 second sprints in search of food.[251,254] The Ache women undergo long periods of activity as well as they spend a large fraction of the day moving camp.[255] As described by Dr. Kim Hill, an anthropologist who has spent much time with the Ache people, "They sprint, jog, climb, carry, jump, etc. all day long." Interestingly and not surprisingly, studies were performed on these same individuals revealing elite physical abilities. The present-day Maasai in Kenya continue to walk extended distances, even though they are part hunter-gatherers, part pastoral.[256]

Unfortunately, under the time constraints of work traditional methods of "exercise" have been replaced by extended periods of sitting at a desk involving little physical activity. To attempt to balance the lack of physical activity and a sedentary workplace, the modern man now engages in compensatory periods of jogging and endurance training.

What Happens to the Body after a Lifetime of Endurance Training?

Those who compete in marathons, triathlons, and other endurance events have been considered the quintessential beings of fitness. Yet, newer data is revealing that the health of these individuals paints a much different picture, one closer to the naked Pheidippides after collapsing, especially when it comes to effects on the heart. In fact, recent data is nearly echoing what Pheidippides showed us some 2,500 years ago, and once again, when the history of humanity is ignored, health suffers. Many physicians are now regularly seeing 50-year-old male joggers with evidence of heart damage and an irregular heartbeat.

Since the heart seems to be the major organ damaged from excessive running, most of the current studies have focused on it. A recent study followed 40 athletes and analyzed several cardiac factors at baseline, after a bout of endurance exercise, and one week later to assess the effects on the heart.[257] The results revealed damage to the right side of the heart, as well as the release of cardiac enzymes, both in direct proportion to race time. Cardiac enzymes are released from the heart when the myocardial cells (muscle cells within the heart) are damaged. The longer the participants trained the more heart damage and dysfunction they experienced. This dysfunction mostly resolved within a week; however, and most importantly, in those participants who chronically engaged in endurance exercise, the muscles in the heart attempted to combat the pounding by becoming hardened and fibrotic, also known as cardiac remodeling.

Extensive studies in runners of the Boston Marathon have analyzed heart function and troponin levels, revealing some remarkable results. Troponin is a protein that is attached to heart muscle and released into the blood stream after severe heart damage. It signals a heart attack when elevated above a certain level.

Echocardiograms were also assessed, which are ultrasound images of the heart. The echocardiograms done in marathon participants revealed more right-sided ventricular heart damage and dysfunction with impaired heart filling as it prepares to pump blood, along with a resulting increased pressure on the lungs, also known as pulmonary pressure.[258] Several biomarkers were increased and over sixty percent of runners had significantly increased troponin levels signifying severe damage to their heart. Astoundingly, forty percent of the runners had such elevated levels of troponin in their blood that, had they presented to the local emergency room, they would have been treated for a heart attack.

Yet, this damage is not only limited to right side of the heart, as studies have shown that prolonged endurance exercise decreases function of the left ventricle as well.[259] A similar study showed that left ventricular dysfunction occurs in triathletes, not just marathon runners.[260] While some have questioned whether this damage only occurs in dedicated athletes, data reveals that while Olympic athletes do fare differently,[261] the damage still occurs in non-Olympic athletes and the common runner. In fact, another studied showed that half of lifelong male athletes, though asymptomatic and appearing healthy, had myocardial fibrosis, which results in a stiff heart that is unable to function optimally.[262] Fibrosis of the heart was significantly associated with the number of marathons, ultra-endurance activity, and number of years spent training.

Marathon running has been shown to result in inflammation of the heart and decreased blood flow to the heart, which may explain why runners have an increased risk of heart damage during the marathon. As the blood flow throughout the heart carries with it a supply of oxygen to fuel the damaged heart muscle and aid in repair, any inhibition of this process could be detrimental to heart health.

Other studies show that running a marathon results in the enlargement of the right atrium and ventricle with associated dysfunction, along with the release of troponin from muscle breakdown and B-type natriuretic peptide.[263] This is, in essence, similar to the lab values that would be found during a heart attack. Stressing the body has been shown to be beneficial in many ways; however, it is difficult to envision that mimicking a heart attack through exercise is advantageous. In fact, excessive stress from exercise has been shown to decrease the body's natural hormonal response as well as to damage the autonomic system.[264] This may also account for several of the heart attack deaths during marathons that are often reported in the media.[265]

Furthermore, injury is not limited to the heart in endurance athletes. While all forms of activity can clearly increase the chance for physical injury, studies have shown that the risk of sustaining an activity-related injury is proportional to the duration of intense physical activity on a weekly basis.[266] It is not surprising that the chronic pounding of endurance exercise wears and tears both the joints and heart. Data confirms this, as over a third of runners are injured per year, with a third of these related to knee injuries, and these risks are associated with increased mileage[267] and time of activity.[268] Similar to heart damage in marathon runners, the total time of extreme activity appears to be crucial, potentially favoring shorter, more intense activities.

What the History of Humanity Reveals regarding Exercise

Throughout the past two million years or so, humans spent a large component of the day in pursuit of food, shelter, and animals. The lifting of heavy objects likely accompanied these activities, as food and supplies needed to be transported and shelter needed to be built. Recent studies have researched whether the stress and pounding of endurance training can be replaced with training that involves intervals of intense activity, such as sprints intermixed with less intense periods, similar to the activities of the Ache people mentioned above and likely similar to the history of most humans. Such a strategy could effectively provide the potential cardiovascular benefits of exercise, while minimizing the joint and heart damage that result from jogging and endurance exercise. Such exercise also limits the main factor for injury – total time of extreme activity. The drastically smaller amount of time one would have to spend to engage in these activities is an added bonus to accommodate the busy lives of many.

A recent study showed improvements in vascular function with interval training, hinting at a possibility that this ancestral method of exercise could provide the cardiovascular benefits of exercise without the ill effects. Sprint interval training showed benefits of muscle health by enhancing its ability to metabolize carbohydrates,[269] which decreased the amount of time they linger in the blood supply, potentially raising insulin and fat production. Other studies confirm these findings, revealing that sprint intervals can provide increased muscle oxidative potential and endurance capacity at a fraction of the time and physical cost of the stress of jogging.[269,270]

In comparing sprinting intervals with continuous running, sprinting appears to significantly increase insulin sensitivity and decrease blood sugar levels versus jogging.[271] Sprinting, but not continuous running, reduced LDL and total cholesterol. However, several other benefits were noted as well.

A common goal of a healthy diet and lifestyle is to build up the body's defenses against free radical attack. This can be done by avoiding excess amounts of carbohydrates in the diet[96,272,273] and reducing inflammation.

High intensity training in animal studies via interval

training, results in an increase in glutathione peroxidase activity, which is a protective compound against free radicals within the body.[274] Yet continuous training, similar to that of a 45-minute jog, does not lead to this heath benefit; comparing this with the fact that chronic endurance activity induces responses and releases chemicals that resemble a heart attack, the benefits become clear.

High intensity training, like interval sprinting, increases the intramuscular amount of mitochondria, the powerhouses of cells. This makes them more efficient and improves exercise performance and the muscles' ability to use carbohydrates for energy in the form of glycogen, instead of storing extra fat.[275] It also increases sirtuin content, which has been shown to extend lifespan in yeast[276] and may be activated by resveratrol in red wine.[277]

While the benefits of exercise on bone health were previously discussed, it is well known that the bones need to undergo heavy resistance as the body responds with increasing bone density to prepare for future resistance. As such, physical exercise decreases bone breakdown and activates bone formation. Conversely, endurance training does not provide this benefit and actually may decrease bone mineral density in the lower spine.[278]

Just like modern diets that are foreign to our bodies and upon which humans cannot thrive, modern exercise is often no different. Injury to the heart and body is not a motive to engage in exercise, and avoiding long duration and endurance training may be the best bet to provide the benefits of exercise, while minimizing damage to the joints and cardiovascular system. An added bonus is the amount of time saved from the abbreviated workouts.

The Benefits of Short Interval, High Intensity Workouts and Heavy Weight Training

1. Saves many hours per week versus jogging and endurance training[270]
2. Increases insulin sensitivity and decreases blood sugar levels over jogging[271]
3. Is more efficient at increasing exercise capacity and aerobic power[279]
4. Provides increased fat loss and better physique[100]
5. Enhances muscle aerobic metabolism[280]
6. Increases testosterone, growth hormone, and IGF-BP,[281] which helps fights cancer, while overtraining disturbs autonomic function[264]
7. Increase strength, explosiveness, and performance[282,283]
8. Reduces wear and tear on joints and ligaments that occurs during long periods of endurance training
9. Results in less neurologic fatigue and risk of injury, i.e. when one reaches neurologic failure from extended training, the joints, tendons and ligaments are recruited to carry the load instead of the muscles, which often results in injury
10. Provides increased muscle mass, decreased body fat, and less muscle wasting that occurs with endurance exercise
11. Leaves the heart more efficient and requiring less oxygen to function well[284]

THE SUN: CAUSING CANCER OR PROVIDING HEALTH?

"There is no evidence that sunscreens protect you from malignant melanoma."
        –United States Environmental Protection Agency

A major public health campaign within the past several decades was undertaken with the goal of reducing the "harmful" effects of the sun. The campaigns varied from the Center for Disease Control's "Choose your Cover" to the "Sunscreen for your Sun Day" campaign. The potential damaging effects of the sun are easily visualized through sunburns and the damaged skin in those with a history of frequent tanning bed usage as well as the leathery skin often seen in Florida retirees.

While it is relatively clearer that sun exposure may lead

to the nearly benign basal cell carcinomas and slightly more aggressive skin squamous cell carcinomas, a contentious question remains: is melanoma risk related to sun exposure? Perhaps more importantly, medicine has failed to ask the question whether the sun actually provides any benefits or even more benefits than risks.

Anecdotally, it is easy to answer this question with both yes and no. To answer yes, one can turn to Australia, a country compiled of a large population of British inhabitants, whose ancestors lived in Western Europe where they received little sun exposure. They now experience abundant sunshine as Australia is an equatorial country with both tropical and desert climates. It also has the highest incidence of melanoma in the world,[285] pointing to the sun as the likely culprit. Conversely, there are accounts of high melanoma rates on parts of the body that never even see the sun. Bob Marley, for example, died of a melanoma on his foot. Some say it was from trauma that the area received during a soccer game. These anecdotal reports provide caution to solely blaming the sun for melanoma.

Sun Exposure and Melanoma

Adding further confusion to the topic is the mixed survival data with sun exposure and melanoma. In European patients diagnosed with melanoma, those with a *higher* frequency of intermittent sun exposure experienced a better survival.[286] Interestingly, an even larger study revealed that melanoma patients with a history of high intermittent sun exposure and skin burns had a decreased risk of dying from their melanomas.[287]

Still other data has revealed that high occupational exposure to the sun results in *less* risk of melanoma,[288] though it is unclear if data like this is simply selecting for areas where sun exposure is more common and the natives are therefore more genetically capable of withstanding increased sun exposure. Along these lines, the countries within Europe that encounter the most annual sunlight have significantly less mortality from melanoma,[289] pointing towards factors other than sunlight leading to death from melanoma and questioning whether sunlight may be providing beneficial aspects that lead to increased survival.

Mechanisms of Damage

Besides the obvious visual damage that the sun can provide after a long day at the beach, a closer look at the mechanism of sun damage is necessary to understand the potential risks and benefits of sun exposure. A plethora of data exist revealing the potentially harmful effects of ultraviolet (UV) radiation. Most data examine the interaction between UV rays and the skin.

UV rays are similar to visible light, but with a significantly shorter wavelength, leaving them invisible to the human eye but able to penetrate the skin. For simplicity, they can be divided into UVA and UVB, as UVC is absorbed by the ozone layer. UVA rays are generally considered the deeply penetrating rays that pass through the ozone layer unscathed and proceed to pass into the deep layers of the skin. They make up around ninety-five percent of the UV rays that humans encounter. They are present during light hours of the day, and can pass through clouds and glass, and as such, humans are exposed to UVA rays year round.

Due to its penetrating properties, UVA is considered the major cause of skin aging, but most consider it less important in skin cancer as it passes through the outermost layer of the skin, known as the epidermis, where skin cancer frequently occurs. UVA exposure results in a significant tanning effect, as it causes the oxidation of melanin, the pigmented component of the skin that lies within the bottom layer of the epidermis, known as the basal layer. As a result, tanning beds are typically made to produce significant amounts of UVA, often over 10 times more than the sun, in order to optimize this reaction and cause the largest amount of skin color change. Similar to the discussion above regarding the oxidation of oils, this process results in the production of free radicals, which can lead to indirect DNA damage.

UVB rays, on the other hand, only partially pass through the ozone layer. UVB is mostly present between the hours of mid-morning and late afternoon and is unable to penetrate glass. As they are less penetrating, they are mostly absorbed in the epidermis of the skin. As a result, UVB rays can typically lead to sun burns and damage to this outer layer of the skin. They also stimulate the synthesis of melanin, leading to increased skin pigment and tanned skin, which provides photo-protection from future sun exposure. Vitamin D production also occurs within the skin from exposure to UVB rays.

Due to their burning potential, methods to limit UVB exposure were at the forefront of the campaign to minimize the potential dangers of the sun by the scientific and medical community. UVB rays provided visual evidence of the potential damage from the sun and thus became an easy target.

Australia had one of the most famous campaigns, known as the "Slip, Slop, Slap, Seek, Slide" campaign, where citizens were told to, "Slip on a shirt, slop on sunscreen, slap on a hat, seek shade, and slide on some sunnies." This campaign was funded through donations and is considered one of the most successful in the world at helping reduce sun exposure, and it is considered by many as the most successful public health campaign in the history of Australia.

The American Cancer Society followed suit with their "Slip! Slop! Slap! And Wrap!" campaign promoting slipping on a shirt, slopping on sunscreen, slapping on a hat, and wrapping on a pair of sunglasses. They also renamed the Friday before Memorial Day as "Don't Fry Day."

These campaigns aimed at sun minimization through direct avoidance by staying indoors or wearing clothing that block the sun, such as shirts or sunglasses. They also promoted methods to limit UVB exposure when in the sun, specifically by applying sunscreens to block the sun's UV rays as well as avoiding the sun between the hours of 10 a.m. and 4 p.m., when UVB rays are at their peak

The campaign to reduce sun exposure was a success in regards to its implementation, but the outcome in regards to cancer rates paints a much different picture. In Australia, rates of the more benign basal cell and squamous cell carcinomas were "slapped" downwards, while the Aussies watched as their rates of the more deadly melanoma skyrocketed. Trends followed in the U.S. as well, as melanoma rates continue to climb and the rates in women have nearly tripled in the past several decades.[290] In fact, between 1973 and 2003, the incidence of melanoma has skyrocketed faster than nearly all other cancers, increasing by over eighty percent.[291] It continues to increase at three percent per year and remains one of the most rapidly increasing cancer diagnoses.

Why the Unexpected Results?

Severe skin burns from prolonged sun exposure as a child have been correlated with an increased risk of melanoma,[292] and other data have revealed that sunburns at any age are correlated with an increased risk of melanoma.[293] Combining data like these along with the knowledge of the damaging effects of the ultraviolet rays of the sun, it seemed without doubt that the medical community had to move fast to remove people from the sun or cover them up with sunblock. However, as is often the case in medicine, correlation does not equal causation and extrapolating from correlative data can often lead to unwanted results.

The data revealing a connection with sunburns and melanoma, combined with the known potential damage of UV rays on the skin naturally lead to the conclusion that avoidance of the sun was a natural step towards reducing the risk of cancer. These steps were considered of extreme importance as 76,690 men and women were diagnosed with melanoma in 2013 alone, and 9,480, or about twelve percent, will die from their disease. While sun exposure has only been correlated with melanoma risk, this correlation, along with preclinical data, have fueled the massive campaign to avoid the sun.

Yet, other data reveals mixed results, and some have even questioned the significance of the positive association between sun exposure and melanoma.[294] Recent data have even revealed that as long as sunburns are kept to a minimum, *increased* sun exposure *decreases* the risk of melanoma.[295] Recent studies have shown a mixed picture regarding sunblock and some have shown an increase in melanoma risk with the usage of sunblock.[296]

Newer data is revealing that UVB also provides the skin with mechanisms for future protection from the sun through tanning, thickening of the skin to increase protection, and the synthesis of vitamin D and melatonin. These factors, with several other unknown factors likely contribute to the beneficial effects of the sun and the potential increase in cancer occurrence with sun avoidance. While direct efforts to avoid sun damage were carried out via UVB-blocking sunscreen and avoidance of the sun during late morning and the afternoon, recent data actually reveal that the indirect oxidative damage of UVA rays may be the main culprit behind increased melanoma risk and not the direct DNA damage of UVB rays. As a result, efforts worked to block UVB rays from contact with the skin, minimizing any potential benefit, leaving the potentially more dangerous UVA rays unchecked.

Skin cancer often occurs in areas that encounter trauma, whether physical trauma or inflammation resulting from sun burns. In fact, Indian women that wear sarees, or garments that wrap around the waist, have been known to experience what is called saree cancer, which is basically cancer that arises along the waist from constant irritation from rubbing of their saree.[297] While sunburn may act in this same regard by irritating the skin, a sunburn and general sun exposure must be differentiated. Avoiding sun burns by removing oneself from direct sun contact after the skin receives its maximum tolerated amount may be an efficacious method of gaining the benefits of the sun while avoiding the potential damaging effects, as vitamin D production is maximal during the first 30-60 minutes of sun exposure.

Cancer and the Sun beyond Melanoma

Digging deeper within the data, several other important facts pertaining to melanoma reveal themselves. First and foremost, out of 100,000 individuals, 21.1 will be diagnosed with melanoma on a yearly basis, or in other words, 0.021%. Overall, one in 49 people will be diagnosed with melanoma in their lifetime. Contrasting these data is the unfortunate fact that breast cancer afflicts one in eight women, while prostate cancer is diagnosed in one of six men. Colon cancer is slightly less prevalent, but well over twice as common as melanoma, with one in 21 men and women experiencing this disease within their lifetime.[298]

While colon and breast cancer are several fold more common than melanoma, they are also more lethal. Overall at five years, ninety-five percent of patients diagnosed with melanoma will be alive. This number drops to eighty-nine percent of breast cancer patients, and survival at five years drops significantly for colon cancer patients with only sixty-five percent of them remaining alive. To sum up these numbers, melanoma remains one of the rarest cancers we experience, with a lower death rate than the more common cancers such as breast and colon cancer.

Yet, while sun exposure may increase the risk of melanoma, and even this data is unclear, it would appear that sun exposure may decrease the risk of the more common breast,[299] prostate,[300] and colon cancer.[301] A closer look at the data also reveals that sunlight exposure may reduce the risk of lung cancer, which is the third most common cancer and one of the most deadly;[302] however, this data specifically reveals a correlation with lower levels of UVB rays and an increased risk of lung cancer in 111 countries.

We aimed to reduce the risk of the least common cancer to potentially increase the risk of the three most common cancers. Unfortunately, it would appear that the major efforts to reduce melanoma risk may have failed or even contributed to its recent increase in prevalence.

While a simple assessment of the numbers reveals potential issues of increasing the ratio of UVA to UVB or total avoidance of the sun, a closer look at the physiologic effects of the sun uncovers at least several of the beneficial health effects of the sun.

The most well-known benefit of the sun is the ability of UVB rays to convert cholesterol to vitamin D within the skin. Vitamin D has many physiologic functions leading to numerous health benefits including improved bone health and the prevention of osteoporosis, cardiovascular health and the reduction of heart disease, insulin function and reduction in the risk of type 1 diabetes. It also supports the immune system to fight infection, autoimmune disease, and cancer.[303]

The benefits of the sun and bone health were realized as far back as 1822, when it was recognized that sun exposure could cure Rickets, a disease characterized by severe bone abnormalities in children.[304] Children with rickets were eventually treated by exposure to a sun lamp to mimic the sun's beneficial rays.

In fact, the body is so genetically adapted to process sun exposure that it is essentially impossible for excessive sun exposure to lead to vitamin D intoxication. When the body encounters prolonged sun exposure, excess vitamin D is destroyed in the skin.[305] However, significant studies exist revealing the recent worldwide surge in vitamin D deficiency.

The recent increase in vitamin D deficiency in Australia has caused the experts to rethink their sun exposure recommendations.[306] Even in Saudi Arabia, one of the sunniest countries in the world, vitamin D deficiency is rampant in the female population due to limited sunlight exposure as women wear burkas.[307] It has also recently been found that UV rays promote the synthesis of melatonin,[308] which provides many antioxidant and anticancer effects throughout the body. Melatonin, a hormone secreted from the brain during sleep, can scavenge free radicals to help prevent cellular damage,[309] it upregulates the immune system to fight inflammation and pathogens, and it even results in suppression of the estrogen receptor gene,[310] which may help prevent and treat breast cancer. It also appears to inhibit several pathways that cancer cells rely upon to stay alive.[311]

Low levels of vitamin D have been associated with increased cancer incidence and mortality in men, setting off a plethora of studies further connecting the two.[312] Postmenopausal women randomized to receive vitamin D experienced a reduction in cancer risk.[313] In a petri dish, when prostate cancer cells are treated with vitamin D3, the proliferation of the cancer cells is inhibited.[314] Another study showed that colorectal cancer rates drop lower as ones vitamin D intake rises.[315] An analysis reviewing nine studies and one million patients revealed that the higher the levels of vitamin D in the blood, the lower the risk of cancer.[316] Interestingly, colon cancer rates are highest in areas of the U.S. where sunlight exposure is the least.[317]

Vitamin D also stimulates the immune system, which helps to fight cancer along with infections. It binds and activates B and T cells, which are the immune system's line of defense against foreign pathogens and infection. Vitamin D has even been used as a treatment for tuberculosis, influenza, and bacterial and viral infections.[318]

Bone health depends on vitamin D levels as well. As described above, studies show that vitamin D levels are the dominant predictor of bone density rather than calcium.[233] It is not surprising that avoidance of the major provider of vitamin D has resulted in decreased levels of this vitamin, along with decreased bone health and increased rates of bone weakness and fractures. Since its highly successful campaign, Australia has experienced a surge in the rates of bone fractures related to osteoporosis, costing their health system an estimated $1.9 billion per year in treatment expenditures. Even financial models have exposed the "cost" of avoiding the sun, as current estimates have revealed that low vitamin D from "inadequate exposure to solar UVB irradiance" is costing the U.S. an estimated $40 to $56 billion, while the price tag of excess sun exposure costs around $6 to $7 billion per year.[319]

Due to the many benefits of vitamin D, some of which currently remain unknown, it is no surprise that low levels are strongly associated with an increase in death from any cause as well as death from cancer, cardiovascular disease, and even respiratory disease.[320] While the sun is a major source of vitamin D, its avoidance should naturally promote acquiring it through food and dietary sources. It is commonly found in whole-fat dairy, meat, and eggs, all foods that have been vilified by the medical field and our governing bodies due to their high-fat content. Vitamin D is also generally found in foods containing large amounts of cholesterol.

Cod liver oil remains as the food with the largest vitamin D content, and it also has one of the highest amounts of cholesterol. With such a large vitamin D content, it was even used to treat childhood bone disease in the 1800s. Not until a century later in the 1900s did scientists realize that the beneficial effects of cod liver oil were largely due to its large vitamin D content. While dietary and even supplementation with vitamin D during times of minimal sun exposure may serve to raise levels within the body, supplementation with vitamin D does not appear to afford the same benefits as sun exposure, revealing that there are likely unknown benefits of the sun that we have yet to realize.[321] Sun exposure also likely contributes to circadian rhythm activation, or appropriate sleep cycles, which leads to further release of cancer-fighting melatonin, among other health benefits. Studies also reveal that chronic sun exposure may provide additional benefits when compared to intermittent exposure, pointing towards other mechanisms as well.

Once again, when referring to the history of humans, most experienced extended periods of sun exposure, whether year round or seasonal. Interestingly and most likely not coincidentally, during the winter months, the human diet would generally rely more heavily on animal sources of sustenance, often high in fat, as plant life was not around. Accompanying this fat was vitamin D. The diet generally consisted of lower sources of fat during the summer months, when plenty of fruits and vegetables were available along with the sun. Basically, when the sun is not present to replenish the body's content of vitamin D, the diet appears to account for this. Avoiding both a high-fat diet and exposure to the sun leaves no possible method of acquiring the physiologically required amounts of vitamin D by the body for healthy bone formation, immune system function, and the ability to fight cancer.

Digging deeper, the adaptations with which the body has acquired to deal with sun exposure further illustrates the importance of sun exposure and health. While the sun's rays activate vitamin D production within the skin, innate physiologic mechanisms are in place to ensure that levels do not rise above toxicity, including degradation when levels become too high. When exposed to unblocked sunlight and UVB rays, the skin can often provide enough vitamin D after only 30 minutes. The process of tanning appears to provide further protection from potential sun damage through methods that are similar to an athlete placing dark pigment under the eyes prior to a game in the sun.[322] Combining all these factors, it seems prudent to get enough sun to stimulate vitamin D production, and then to seek out shade to avoid photodamage or sunburns. Tanning appears to provide future protection as well. Strictly avoiding the sun may put one in a much worse position than getting slightly too much sun, though no current studies have addressed this issue. Using sun lotion to block out UVB rays may be worse yet. However, as is often the case in all aspects of health and wellness, taking a polarizing view often leaves one incapable of visualizing the other health-promoting aspects that may be right under the sun.

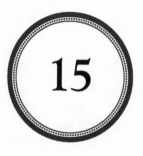

SALT

"The cure for anything is salt water:
sweat, tears or the sea."
–Isak Dinesen,
winner of the Nobel Prize in literature

Salt has had a large presence within humanity from the dawn of time, distinguishing itself as a staple of the human diet. Jesus referred to his followers as the salt of the earth, paying homage to the importance of salt in the human diet. Sabbath bread is dipped into salt to preserve the covenant with God in Judaism. Muhammad described four blessings sent down by God: iron, fire, water, and salt. Within the history of humanity, the health benefits of salt have been known for centuries. Yet, humans are not the only species to rely on salt for survival.

Elephants, buffalo, and even hyenas will travel extensive distances to obtain salt. In Kenya, elephants will travel deep into the Kitum Cave risking death and injury to mine its salt deposits.[323] These elephants risk death by falling into the deep crevasses along the trail as well as being hunted by predators. Since salt is such a vital necessity for life, these elephants brave the journey to obtain it.

Fast-forwarding two million years or so, the dietary restriction of salt has been a stalwart recommendation by health officials for several decades in an attempt to lower blood pressure and avoid heart disease.[324] The commonly cited reason for salt restriction is due to its potential increase in blood pressure, though the belief that salt negatively affects general health often resonates within the medical community. The Japanese, who have the highest salt intake in the world are often believed to be one of the healthiest societies around the globe with the longest longevity and appear to disagree with these recommendations.[325] As is often the case with healthcare and dietary advice, there is a plethora of conflicting epidemiologic data with some showing that a high salt intake, especially in the face of the carbohydrate-laden standard American diet, may be detrimental to health. Other data does not support such conclusions.

The Studies

As there is an enormous amount of conflicting studies, several large analyses have been conducted to sort through the rubble. In essence, these studies combine individual studies to assess the outcome in terms of the larger picture. One such assessment revealed a decrease in systolic blood pressure of five mmHg in those with high blood pressure and two mmHg in those with normal blood pressure. Considering a normal blood pressure is 120/80 (i.e. systolic 120 and diastolic 80), these changes were infinitesimally small and likely irrelevant.

However, these changes were considered significant in the analysis due to the large number of individuals included, as 734 individuals with elevated blood pressure and 2,220 with normal blood pressure were assessed.[326] The conclusion of this study was that salt reduction is an effective method of reducing blood pressure. Another study in patients with prehypertension revealed that salt restriction may decrease cardiovascular events, such as heart attacks; however, there was no significant change in mortality with modifying salt intake.[327]

On the other hand, another much larger and more extensive meta-analysis assessed 57 trials including 5,030 individuals, finding that a low-sodium diet reduced blood pressure by only one percent. The authors even concluded that these findings do not support recommendations to consume less sodium.[328] This should provide caution in reducing a physiologically necessary nutrient such as salt. Still, such data is generally overlooked or even ignored.

Nevertheless, if changes in blood pressure alone, regardless of how minor, do not lead to changes in mortality, one has to question whether it is prudent to alter a behavior. This becomes especially important if this change does not actually result in a different outcome regarding lifespan or even overall health. Several studies observing salt intake and death have taken place to answer this question.

Recently, European researchers have evaluated whether 24-hour urine sodium excretion predicts blood pressure and mortality.[329] They used urinary secretion as a marker for sodium intake in the diet, which is considered the most accurate assessment of salt intake (i.e. the more salt consumed, the more excreted in the urine). The prospective study involved 3,681 participants over twenty years, 2,096 of whom had normal blood pressure. The researchers found that lower sodium consumption was associated with *higher* cardiovascular death. In other words, the less salt one ate the greater chance of cardiovascular death. While some studies may show a minor decrease in blood pressure, such changes are insignificant if death rate is increased. In fact, such changes may be outright harmful. This study holds increased importance for those who do not have elevated blood pressure and are merely trying to construct the healthiest diet and lifestyle possible.

The National Health and Nutrition Examination Survey (NHANES) reported on three massive studies analyzing sodium intake and mortality in thousands of individuals. However, the study evaluated sodium intake relying on dietary recall, which is fraught with error and bias and likely less accurate than measuring urinary levels. Regardless, these are some of the largest studies undertaken that assess salt intake and mortality. The results were as follows:

1. NHANES I revealed a decrease in cardiovascular and all-cause mortality, or dying from any cause, with *increased* salt consumption.[330]
2. NHANES II revealed similar findings that increased salt consumption led to a *decrease* in cardiovascular disease mortality with the highest risk in those that limited their sodium to fewer than 2300mg per day.[331]
3. NHANES III showed similar, but statistically non-significant increases in mortality with lower sodium consumption.[332]

Three of the largest studies ever undertaken revealed *detrimental* outcomes with extreme salt restriction. Even recent data in patients with congestive heart failure, whom often experience fluid overload and swelling, have shown that a reduced salt diet results in increased hospitalizations and worse clinical outcomes.[333] Patients with diabetes may not fare differently as studies have revealed that diabetics with decreased sodium consumption experience increased all-cause and cardiovascular mortality.[334]

Regardless, the topic of salt restriction remains one of stark controversy. While epidemiologic data shows that salt intake may raise blood pressure, many studies have revealed that lowering salt intake below recommended levels may have the opposite effect by increasing the risk of death.

The Physiologic Function of Salt

Sodium from salt is a vital nutrient within the diet. Table salt is forty percent sodium and sixty percent chloride. Sodium helps the body maintain cellular water balance, blood volume, and pH. It is also vital in neuron, or nerve cell, functioning by supporting the transport of nerve impulses from the brain to the muscles, resulting in contractions. When blood pressure or the blood's concentration of sodium decreases, the renin-angiotensin system calls upon the kidneys to absorb more sodium, decreasing the amount lost in the urine. As a result, low dietary sodium causes the body to release several potentially harmful hormones like renin, aldosterone, and noradrenaline to compensate.[335] Sodium in the diet has the opposite effect, pulling water with it and thus supporting the circulatory system. This is also why the overconsumption of salt may lead to an increase in swelling in some individuals.

Sodium supports the circulatory system, and animal studies show that a low-salt diet leads to higher susceptibility of cardiovascular collapse and impaired ability to adjust to stress.[336] In other words, sodium pulls water into the blood allowing the circulatory system to function to its fullest while keeping fluid within the body. Dietary sodium largely comes into play for circulatory support, especially in those who exercise often and lose a significant amount of sodium through perspiration. Along these lines, studies show that vigorous exercise for one hour in hot weather can result in salt loss that exceeds the recommended daily allowance.[337] Such data would favor a much higher intake of sodium in athletes or those that work out vigorously or frequently, and in these populations salt restriction may be even more dangerous.

What Causes the Kidneys to Retain Salt?

Much like calcium and bone strength, the issue of sodium content in the body is not merely a factor of salt intake. As discussed above, the renal-angiotensin system regulates the reabsorption and excretion of salt based on the commands it receives from the body. The body's sodium levels are based on a delicate interplay between salt intake in the diet and sodium lost through the kidneys via urine, through sweat, and in the GI tract, along with hormones that act on the kidney.

Much like with calcium and many other minerals and electrolytes in the diet, the kidney is the gatekeeper, constantly hard at work filtering our blood and keeping some substances in, or reabsorbing them, and secreting others with the urine. Viewing sodium as an in versus out equation, much like calcium and calories, is shortsighted and incorrect. Insulin, the hormone within the body that is secreted by the pancreas to lower blood sugar after a carbohydrate-rich meal, directly signals the kidney to reabsorb sodium.[338]

In fact, when individuals are given exogenous insulin, a signal is almost immediately sent to the kidneys to stop secreting sodium in the urine and to send it back into the blood supply. Along these lines, carbohydrate intake leads to both an increase in blood sugar and insulin, resulting in significant retention of sodium within the kidneys.[339] Once again insulin adds fuel to the fire, and methods to minimize insulin levels may benefit health in this regard. It would appear that salt is merely collateral damage in many of our current dietary recommendations that are based on a food that causes the kidneys to retain sodium, falsely putting the blame on sodium within the diet.

Interestingly, it is well known within the diet and nutrition world that when individuals pursue a low-carbohydrate diet, they often experience fluid loss. When insulin drops from low levels of carbohydrates within the diet, it allows the kidneys to stop retaining as much sodium, therefore pulling fluid into the urine leading to water loss.

Not only do increased carbohydrates in the diet lead to elevated levels of insulin and sodium retention, but studies show that low-salt diets actually inhibit the ability of insulin to lower blood glucose levels and can actually lead to insulin resistance.[340] This results in increased levels of circulating insulin and a physiologic state resembling that of a diabetic. Animal studies confirm this, revealing that a low salt diet in rats leads to increased fat accumulation throughout the body and insulin resistance.[341] Even a moderate reduction of salt can negatively impact insulin sensitivity, and another study reveals that it "aggravates both systemic and vascular insulin resistance."[342]

Perhaps this is one reason why low salt intake was associated with increased death rates in diabetics.[334] While decreased salt intake has been shown to raise blood sugar levels, it has also been shown to activate the sympathetic nervous system,[343] known as the fight or flight response, thus raising levels of chronic stress. Ironically, reducing salt has also been shown to raise LDL, the so-called "bad cholesterol," and overall cholesterol,[335] going directly against the goal of recommendations by conventional wisdom to lower cholesterol.

Studies of a High-Fat, Low-Carbohydrate Diet

In a study comparing a low-fat, calorie-reduced diet versus a low-carbohydrate diet with no restriction of calories, participants on the low-carbohydrate study were instructed to drink bouillon dissolved in water two to three times per day,[344] which roughly correlates to one to two grams of sodium. Knowing that a low-carbohydrate diet will decrease insulin significantly and therefore lead to loss of sodium from the kidneys, the scientists preemptively raised the participants' salt intake. While they significantly increased their salt intake, their systolic blood pressure dropped by 17 points and diastolic dropped by eight. This can partly be explained by the improved metabolic status of these individuals on a reduced carbohydrate diet, including weight loss, decreased blood glucose, and decreased insulin. However, this study may further illustrate the fact that when carbohydrate sources of food are not over-consumed, sodium intake may be irrelevant or may even need to be *increased*.

Is the Whole Foods and Low-Carbohydrate Movement Compatible with Lowering Salt Intake?

With the advent of the whole foods movement, along with its subsidiaries, which often include low-carb lifestyles, "paleo," and "caveman" dieting, the consumption of processed foods has fallen drastically in these groups. As a result, salt consumption has also dropped dramatically, as processed foods contain high levels of sodium. When one makes a switch to lower amounts of dietary carbohydrates and reduces the consumption of grains and sugar, blood insulin levels naturally drop as well. As a result, the kidney begins to secrete more sodium into the urine. This is often why low-carb advocates feel run down when they switch to a low-carb lifestyle.

When exercise is added, the problem is compounded, as it often results in significant fluid and sodium loss, further adding to the net negative balance. Drinking excess fluid to replace the lost volume in sweat, may further dilute the salt balance resulting in hyponatremia (low blood sodium levels),[345] which can result in serious consequences.

Once again, returning to the history of humans, over the past 2.5 million years, the human diet consisted of mostly wild game, often raw with a significant amount of blood. Some cultures even consume pure blood, though this is rarely seen nowadays. This practice still exists in many traditional diets, including concoctions such as blood pudding, often a part of traditional southern Italian cuisine. The organs and blood of animals contain high amounts of sodium that are not present in the cooked muscle meat. Therefore, it becomes clearer as to why a whole food diet would need supplemented with sodium as the most salt-rich parts of the animal are often no longer consumed as was customary in the past.

For instance, the Maasai of Africa eat around three grams of salt per day,[346] mostly from their intake of whole blood, yet have very low blood pressure. Americans eat about 3.4 grams of sodium per day mostly in the form of processed table salt, which correlates to roughly double the amount of salt.[347] However, the Maasai eat a diet rich in animal meat, blood, and milk that is often fermented, which breaks down the sugar products, leaving a small fraction of the insulin-stimulating carbohydrates that dominate most American's diets. As a result, they have less insulin signaling to their kidneys to retain sodium.

The American Heart Association recommends limiting sodium to less than 1,500 milligrams per day, or roughly four grams of salt, though evidence on this approach and the health benefits and safety have been called "weak, heterogeneous, inconclusive and inconsistent" by critics.[348] Furthermore, recent information from the National Academy of Sciences reveals that some of the authorities are beginning to back away from previous recommendations of excessively limiting sodium as it clearly has negative health effects.[349]

Final Thoughts: Are All Salts the Same?

Like nearly all processed and factory created foods, natural salt and produced salt are quite different. The white table salt that is commonly encountered is refined and processed, which removes trace minerals. Much like in vegetable oils, refining is generally an unhealthy step in food preparation.

After this salt is refined, several chemicals are added including aluminum, ammonium, and ferrocyanide to minimize congealing of the salt and to extend shelf life. In essence, the resulting compound is sodium with several chemicals and often iodine.

Himalayan and natural sea salts are markedly different as they naturally contain several minerals if unrefined. They are not comparable to the factory made, chemically-laden white salt, as they have trace minerals. These minerals have important health implications as data suggests that increasing the intake of salts with more potassium and magnesium may actually lower blood pressure.[350] It is worth mentioning that all studies analyzing salt intake are likely assessing the consumption of salt in the form of processed table salt or processed foods that contain processed salt. If these studies assessed mineral-dense salt, a different picture would likely be painted.

The dietary recommendations to reduce salt once again go against the history of human dietary consumption and are likely catering to the erroneous dietary recommendations of the food pyramid, which lead to an abnormal physiologic state within the body that leads to inappropriate sodium retention. Reducing salt in the diet without fixing the actual problem may cause additional health issues. The consumption of a healthy diet that favors nutrient-dense foods may not only require avoiding recommendations for salt limitation, but may require an increase in salt intake, especially with exercise.

Salt

1. Reducing sodium in the diet minimally affects blood pressure.
2. Reducing sodium in the diet may increase cardiovascular death and death from all causes, especially in average weight and healthy individuals.
3. Low-salt diets may lead to decreased insulin sensitivity and increased fat accumulation throughout the body.
4. A low-carbohydrate lifestyle results in less circulating insulin, causing the kidneys to secrete more sodium in the urine.
5. Strenuous exercise can result in a loss of sodium greater than the recommended daily allowance.
6. Those who exercise often and follow a generally lower carbohydrate lifestyle may want to reconsider recommendations to reduce their sodium intake.
7. Refined table salt is markedly inferior to mineral-rich Himalayan salt or natural sea salt.

CLOSING

"*No disease that can be treated by diet should be treated with any other means.*"

–Maimonides

*T*he history of health reveals the clear pattern of how one improper recommendation can lead to multiple incorrect recommendations and a massive domino effect. It becomes clear that we must strive to take control of our own health and blindly following improper recommendations that change on a daily basis can lead to serious health issues. Physicians can aid us when health goes awry and provide guidance to achieve optimal health, but true optimal heath undoubtedly lies within an individual.

The most effective method of achieving optimal health is by channeling the intrinsic methods that the body has developed during its millions of years on Earth. Recommendations that drastically diverge from this pattern will likely lead to poorer health as has been witnessed over the past three decades.

While it is easy to assign the blame to the modern day physician, one must remember the extreme commitment such a profession demands. Most physicians work exceedingly long hours, often on call at inopportune times pulling them from their family. Most do not have time to research and investigate every finite detail taught during training of follow along with the frequently changing data. As a result, they rely on the recommendations from the medical organizations and governing bodies. Unfortunately, these recommendations are often not based on sound data, or as in the case of the Mc-Govern Committee, there is a complete lack of consensus between the experts regarding these recommendations.

Also, this work is not necessarily meant to be a criticism of all of these campaigns, and it must be remembered that many, if not most, set out to improve the health of our people. The skin cancer prevention campaign had clear implications to decrease a potentially preventable cancer. The marathon and jogging movement seemed like an obvious push for health. However, when a total historical approach is taken, the potential problems become apparent as cancer rates increase with sun avoidance and heart damage accumulates in our population of runners.

The goal of this critical look at medical recommendations is to help the reader bring his or her health back into his or her own hands. We all must take a critical look at our health. We must remember that achieving optimal health includes accomplishing health throughout the entire body. Preventing a heart attack is worthless if one gets cancer in the process, and avoiding melanoma is useless if in doing so, it results in a much more malignant cancer. Reducing sodium may result in a lower blood pressure, but this is meaningless if it results in an increased risk of death or diabetes.

Unfortunately poor recommendations based on nonexistent or insufficient data are often times perpetuated instead of rescinded, leading to further collateral damage. This perpetuation often occurs by nonmedical sources such as the media or special interest groups. For instance, recommending a high carbohydrate diet leads to weight gain and salt retention by the kidneys and therefore false recommendations to limit salt are born. When people are told to avoid the sun and fatty foods, both potent sources of vitamin D, bone health suffers. Instead of pulling back these recommendations, we prescribe calcium, and watch as studies show an increase in mortality from excess calcium supplementation.

Covering up poor recommendations with additional poor recommendations only leads to further health issues. And for this reason the history of human health must be analyzed with each step of this process to ask the question as to whether these recommendations could possibly be healthy or are even rational when viewed historically. The inadequacy of the basis for many of these recommendations becomes quite clear when reviewing the data. However, with the information age upon us, these data are becoming clearer to the general population and in medicine, and studies are underway to reexamine many of these issues. Hopefully this time around, we remember our history as we set out to define our health.

REFERENCES:

1. Prasad V CAIJA. Reversals of established medical practices: Evidence to abandon ship. JAMA: The Journal of the American Medical Association. 2012;307(1):37-38.
2. Ioannidis JPA. Why Most Published Research Findings Are False. PLoS Med. 2005;2(8):e124.
3. Ioannidis JA. Contradicted and initially stronger effects in highly cited clinical research. JAMA: The Journal of the American Medical Association. 2005;294(2):218-228.
4. Heini AF, Weinsier RL. Divergent trends in obesity and fat intake patterns: The american paradox. The American journal of medicine. 1997;102(3):259-264.
5. Cite Centers for Disease Control and Prevention, The Obesity Epidemic. Available at: < http://www.cdc.gov/cdctv/ObesityEpidemic/>. Accessed July 27, 2011
6. CDC. Trends in Intake of Energy and Macronutrients - United States, 1971-2000. 2004; http://www.cdc.gov/mmwr/preview/mmwrhtml/mm5304a3.htm.
7. Konstantinov IE, Mejevoi N, Anichkov NM. Nikolai N. Anichkov and his theory of atherosclerosis. Texas Heart Institute journal / from the Texas Heart Institute of St. Luke's Episcopal Hospital, Texas Children's Hospital. 2006;33(4):417-423.
8. Matrai K. AV, Hahn I. Seasonal diet of rabbits and their browsing effect on juniper in Bugac Juniper Forest (Hungary). Acta Theriologica. 1998;43(1):107-112.
9. Martins H, Milne JA, Rego F. Seasonal and spatial variation in the diet of the wild rabbit (Oryctolagus cuniculus L.) in Portugal. Journal of Zoology. 2002;258(03):395-404.
10. Reddiex B. Diet selection of European rabbits (Oryctola-

gus cuniculus) in the semi-arid grasslands of the Mackenzie Basin, New Zealand: Department of Ecology, Lincoln University; 1998.

11. Wilson R, Miller R, Middleton C, Kinden D. Atherosclerosis in rabbits fed a low cholesterol diet for five years. Arteriosclerosis, Thrombosis, and Vascular Biology. May 1, 1982 1982;2(3):228-241.

12. Minick CR, Murphy GE. Experimental induction of atheroarteriosclerosis by the synergy of allergic injury to arteries and lipid-rich diet. II. Effect of repeatedly injected foreign protein in rabbits fed a lipid-rich, cholesterol-poor diet. The American journal of pathology. Nov 1973;73(2):265-300.

13. Staprans I, Pan X-M, Rapp JH, Feingold KR. Oxidized Cholesterol in the Diet Accelerates the Development of Aortic Atherosclerosis in Cholesterol-Fed Rabbits. Arteriosclerosis, Thrombosis, and Vascular Biology. June 1, 1998 1998;18(6):977-983.

14. Xiu RJ, Freyschuss A, Ying X, Berglund L, Henriksson P, Bjorkhem I. The antioxidant butylated hydroxytoluene prevents early cholesterol-induced microcirculatory changes in rabbits. The Journal of clinical investigation. Jun 1994;93(6):2732-2737.

15. Mahfouz M, Kawano H, Kummerow F. Effect of cholesterol-rich diets with and without added vitamins E and C on the severity of atherosclerosis in rabbits. The American journal of clinical nutrition. November 1, 1997 1997;66(5):1240-1249.

16. Kritchevsky D. History of Recommendations to the Public about Dietary Fat. The Journal of nutrition. February 1, 1998 1998;128(2):449S-452S.

17. Akerblom JL, Costa R, Luchsinger JA, et al. Relation of plasma lipids to all-cause mortality in Caucasian, African-American and Hispanic elders. Age and Ageing. March 1, 2008 2008;37(2):207-213.

18. Kalm LM, Semba RD. They Starved So That Others Be Better Fed: Remembering Ancel Keys and the Minnesota Experiment. The Journal of Nutrition. June 1, 2005 2005;135(6):1347-1352.

19. Keys A. Seven Countries: A Multivariate Analysis of Death and Coronary Heart Disease.: Harvard University Press; 1980.

20. Keys A. Atherosclerosis: a problem in newer public health. Journal of the Mount Sinai Hospital, New York. Jul-Aug 1953;20(2):118-139.

21. Keys A. Coronary heart disease in seven countries. 1970. Nutrition. Mar 1997;13(3):250-252; discussion 249, 253.

22. Yerushalmy J, Hilleboe HE. Fat in the diet and mortality from heart disease; a methodologic note. New York state journal of medicine. 1957;57(14):2343-2354.

23. Castelli WP. Concerning the possibility of a nut. Archives of internal medicine. 1992;152(7):1371-1372.

24. Landé K. E. SWM. Human atherosclerosis in relation to the cholesterol content of the blood. Arch. Pathol. 1936;22:201-312.

25. Mathur KS, Patney NL, Kumar V, Sharma RD. Serum Cholesterol and Atherosclerosis in Man. Circulation. June 1, 1961 1961;23(6):847-852.

26. Paterson JC, Dyer L, Armstrong EC. Serum cholesterol levels in human atherosclerosis. Canadian Medical Association journal. Jan 2 1960;82:6-11.

27. Marek Z, Jaegermann K, Ciba T. Atherosclerosis and levels of serum cholesterol in postmortem investigations. American heart journal. Jun 1962;63:768-774.

28. Cabin HS, Roberts WC. Relation of serum total cholesterol and triglyceride levels to the amount and extent of coronary arterial narrowing by atherosclerotic plaque in coronary heart disease. Quantitative analysis of 2,037 five mm segments of 160 major epicardial coronary arteries in 40 necropsy patients. The American journal of

medicine. Aug 1982;73(2):227-234.

29. Relationship of Atherosclerosis in Young Men to Serum Lipoprotein Cholesterol Concentrations and Smoking. JAMA: The Journal of the American Medical Association. December 19, 1990 1990;264(23):3018-3024.

30. Hecht HS, Harman SM. Relation of aggressiveness of lipid-lowering treatment to changes in calcified plaque burden by electron beam tomography. The American journal of cardiology. Aug 1 2003;92(3):334-336.

31. Brehm BJ, Seeley RJ, Daniels SR, D'Alessio DA. A randomized trial comparing a very low carbohydrate diet and a calorie-restricted low fat diet on body weight and cardiovascular risk factors in healthy women. The Journal of clinical endocrinology and metabolism. Apr 2003;88(4):1617-1623.

32. Gardner CD, Kiazand A, Alhassan S, et al. Comparison of the Atkins, Zone, Ornish, and Learn diets for change in weight and related risk factors among overweight premenopausal women: the A TO Z Weight Loss Study: a randomized trial. JAMA : the journal of the American Medical Association. Mar 7 2007;297(9):969-977.

33. Samaha FF, Iqbal N, Seshadri P, et al. A low-carbohydrate as compared with a low-fat diet in severe obesity. The New England journal of medicine. May 22 2003;348(21):2074-2081.

34. Seshadri P, Iqbal N, Stern L, et al. A randomized study comparing the effects of a low-carbohydrate diet and a conventional diet on lipoprotein subfractions and C-reactive protein levels in patients with severe obesity. The American journal of medicine. Sep 15 2004;117(6):398-405.

35. Shai I, Schwarzfuchs D, Henkin Y, et al. Weight loss with a low-carbohydrate, Mediterranean, or low-fat diet. The New England journal of medicine. Jul 17 2008;359(3):229-241.

36. Stern L, Iqbal N, Seshadri P, et al. The effects of low-carbohydrate versus conventional weight loss diets in severely obese adults: one-year follow-up of a randomized trial. Annals of internal medicine. May 18 2004;140(10):778-785.

37. Yancy WS, Jr., Olsen MK, Guyton JR, Bakst RP, Westman EC. A low-carbohydrate, ketogenic diet versus a low-fat diet to treat obesity and hyperlipidemia: a randomized, controlled trial. Annals of internal medicine. May 18 2004;140(10):769-777.

38. McMichael AJ, Jensen OM, Parkin DM, Zaridze DG. Dietary and endogenous cholesterol and human cancer. Epidemiologic reviews. 1984;6:192-216.

39. Asfaw B, White T, Lovejoy O, Latimer B, Simpson S, Suwa G. Australopithecus garhi: a new species of early hominid from Ethiopia. Science. Apr 23 1999;284(5414):629-635.

40. Rindos D. The Origins of Agriculture: An Evolutionary Perspective: Academic Press; 1987.

41. Pielou EC. After the Ice Age: The Return of Life to Glaciated North America: The University of Chicago Press; 1991.

42. Eaton SB. The ancestral human diet: what was it and should it be a paradigm for contemporary nutrition? The Proceedings of the Nutrition Society. Feb 2006;65(1):1-6.

43. Kannel WB GT. The Framingham Diet Study: diet and the regulations of serum cholesterol (Sect 24). Washington DC: Dept of Health, Education and Welfare; 1970.

44. Nichols AB, Ravenscroft C, Lamphiear DE, Ostrander LD. Independence of Serum Lipid Levels and Dietary Habits. JAMA: The Journal of the American Medical Association. October 25, 1976 1976;236(17):1948-1953.

45. Van Gaal LF, Mertens IL, De Block CE. Mechanisms linking obesity with cardiovascular disease. Nature. 2006;444(7121):875-880.

46. Kannel WB, McGee DL. Diabetes and Cardiovascular

Disease. JAMA: The Journal of the American Medical Association. May 11, 1979 1979;241(19):2035-2038.

47. D Maxwell P. Global cancer statistics in the year 2000. The Lancet Oncology. 2001;2(9):533-543.

48. Foster GD, Wyatt HR, Hill JO, et al. A randomized trial of a low-carbohydrate diet for obesity. The New England journal of medicine. May 22 2003;348(21):2082-2090.

49. Hite AH, Berkowitz VG, Berkowitz K. Low-carbohydrate diet review: shifting the paradigm. Nutr Clin Pract. Jun 2011;26(3):300-308.

50. Wakley T. The Lancet: A Journal of British and Foreign Medical and Chemical Science, Criticism, Literature and News Vol Volume I. London: John Churchill; 1845.

51. Tolstoy L, FitzLyon K. Anna Karenina. Oxford: Oneworld Classics; 2008.

52. Osler W. The Principles and Practive of Medicine. Fourth ed. New York: D. Appleton and Company; 1901.

53. Davidson B, Maciver J, Lessard E, Connors K. Meat Lipid Profiles: A Comparison of Meat from Domesticated and Wild Southern African Animals. In Vivo. March-April 2011 2011;25(2):197-202.

54. Rule DC, Broughton KS, Shellito SM, Maiorano G. Comparison of muscle fatty acid profiles and cholesterol concentrations of bison, beef cattle, elk, and chicken. Journal of Animal Science. May 1, 2002 2002;80(5):1202-1211.

55. Realini CE, Duckett SK, Brito GW, Dalla Rizza M, De Mattos D. Effect of pasture vs. concentrate feeding with or without antioxidants on carcass characteristics, fatty acid composition, and quality of Uruguayan beef. Meat Science. 2004;66(3):567-577.

56. Bulatao E, Carlson AJ. Contributions to the Physiology of the Stomach: Influence of Experimental Changes in Blood Sugar Level on Gastric Hunger Contractions. American Journal of Physiology ~ Legacy Content. June

1, 1924 1924;69(1):107-115.

57. Janowitz HD, Ivy AC. Role of Blood Sugar Levels in Spontaneous and Insulin-Induced Hunger in Man. Journal of Applied Physiology. March 1, 1949 1949;1(9):643-645.

58. Geiselman PJ, Novin D. The role of carbohydrates in appetite, hunger and obesity. Appetite;Appetite. 1982;3(3):203-223.

59. Kahn SE, Hull RL, Utzschneider KM. Mechanisms linking obesity to insulin resistance and type 2 diabetes. Nature. Dec 14 2006;444(7121):840-846.

60. Volek JS, Sharman MJ, Love DM, et al. Body composition and hormonal responses to a carbohydrate-restricted diet. Metabolism: clinical and experimental. 2002;51(7):864-870.

61. Weigle DS, Breen PA, Matthys CC, et al. A high-protein diet induces sustained reductions in appetite, ad libitum caloric intake, and body weight despite compensatory changes in diurnal plasma leptin and ghrelin concentrations. The American journal of clinical nutrition. July 1, 2005 2005;82(1):41-48.

62. Apolzan JW, Carnell NS, Mattes RD, Campbell WW. Inadequate Dietary Protein Increases Hunger and Desire to Eat in Younger and Older Men. The Journal of nutrition. June 1, 2007 2007;137(6):1478-1482.

63. Holt SH, Miller JB. Increased insulin responses to ingested foods are associated with lessened satiety. Appetite. Feb 1995;24(1):43-54.

64. Pennington AW. Treatment of Obesity with Calorically Unrestricted Diets. The American Journal of Clinical Nutrition. July 1, 1953 1953;1(5):343-348.

65. Avena NM, Hoebel BG. A diet promoting sugar dependency causes behavioral cross-sensitization to a low dose of amphetamine. Neuroscience. 2003;122(1):17-20.

66. Avena NM, Rada P, Hoebel BG. Evidence for sugar ad-

diction: Behavioral and neurochemical effects of intermittent, excessive sugar intake. Neuroscience & Biobehavioral Reviews. 2008;32(1):20-39.

67. Colantuoni C, Schwenker J, McCarthy J, et al. Excessive sugar intake alters binding to dopamine and mu-opioid receptors in the brain. NeuroReport. 2001;12(16):3549-3552.

68. Rada P, Avena NM, Hoebel BG. Daily bingeing on sugar repeatedly releases dopamine in the accumbens shell. Neuroscience. 2005;134(3):737-744.

69. Lustig RH, Rose SR, Burghen GA, et al. Hypothalamic obesity caused by cranial insult in children: Altered glucose and insulin dynamics and reversal by a somatostatin agonist. The Journal of Pediatrics. 1999;135(2):162-168.

70. Mehran Arya E, Templeman Nicole M, Brigidi GS, et al. Hyperinsulinemia Drives Diet-Induced Obesity Independently of Brain Insulin Production. Cell metabolism. 2012;16(6):723-737.

71. Hite AH, Berkowitz VG, Berkowitz K. Low-carbohydrate diet review: shifting the paradigm. Nutrition in clinical practice : official publication of the American Society for Parenteral and Enteral Nutrition. Jun 2011;26(3):300-308.

72. Booth DA, Chase A, Campbell AT. Relative effectiveness of protein in the late stages of appetite suppression in man. Physiology & Behavior. 1970;5(11):1299-1302.

73. Hargrove JL. History of the Calorie in Nutrition. The Journal of nutrition. December 2006 2006;136(12):2957-2961.

74. Phinney SD, LaGrange BM, O'Connell M, Danforth Jr E. Effects of aerobic exercise on energy expenditure and nitrogen balance during very low calorie dieting. Metabolism. 1988;37(8):758-765.

75. Ebbeling Cb SJFFHA, et al. Effects of dietary composition on energy expenditure during weight-loss main-

tenance. JAMA: The Journal of the American Medical Association. 2012;307(24):2627-2634.

76. Cirillo D, Rachiglio AM, la Montagna R, Giordano A, Normanno N. Leptin signaling in breast cancer: an overview. Journal of cellular biochemistry. Nov 1 2008;105(4):956-964.

77. Fantuzzi G, Faggioni R. Leptin in the regulation of immunity, inflammation, and hematopoiesis. J Leukoc Biol. Oct 2000;68(4):437-446.

78. Friedman JM, Halaas JL. Leptin and the regulation of body weight in mammals. Nature. 1998;395(6704):763-770.

79. Garofalo C, Surmacz E. Leptin and cancer. Journal of cellular physiology. Apr 2006;207(1):12-22.

80. Hekerman P, Zeidler J, Korfmacher S, et al. Leptin induces inflammation-related genes in RINm5F insulinoma cells. BMC Molecular Biology. 2007;8(1):41.

81. Goodwin PJ, Ennis M, Pritchard KI, et al. Fasting insulin and outcome in early-stage breast cancer: results of a prospective cohort study. Journal of clinical oncology : official journal of the American Society of Clinical Oncology. Jan 1 2002;20(1):42-51.

82. Jaggers JR, Sui X, Hooker SP, et al. Metabolic syndrome and risk of cancer mortality in men. Eur J Cancer. 2009;45(10):1831-1838.

83. Kanety H, Madjar Y, Dagan Y, et al. Serum insulin-like growth factor-binding protein-2 (IGFBP-2) is increased and IGFBP-3 is decreased in patients with prostate cancer: correlation with serum prostate-specific antigen. Journal of Clinical Endocrinology & Metabolism. July 1, 1993 1993;77(1):229-233.

84. Pollak M. Insulin, insulin-like growth factors and neoplasia. Best Pract Res Clin Endocrinol Metab. Aug 2008;22(4):625-638.

85. Sachdev D, Yee D. The IGF system and breast cancer.

Endocr Relat Cancer. Sep 2001;8(3):197-209.

86. Freiberg JJ, Tybjærg-Hansen A, Jensen JS, Nordestgaard BG. Nonfasting Triglycerides and Risk of Ischemic Stroke in the General Population. JAMA: The Journal of the American Medical Association. November 12, 2008 2008;300(18):2142-2152.

87. Goodwin PJ, Boyd NF, Hanna W, et al. Elevated levels of plasma triglycerides are associated with histologically defined premenopausal breast cancer risk. Nutrition and cancer. 1997;27(3):284-292.

88. Hokanson JE, Austin MA. Plasma triglyceride level is a risk factor for cardiovascular disease independent of high-density lipoprotein cholesterol level: a meta-analysis of population-based prospective studies. Journal of cardiovascular risk. Apr 1996;3(2):213-219.

89. Foekens JA, Schmitt M, van Putten WL, et al. Plasminogen activator inhibitor-1 and prognosis in primary breast cancer. Journal of Clinical Oncology. August 1, 1994 1994;12(8):1648-1658.

90. Landin K, Stigendal L, Eriksson E, et al. Abdominal obesity is associated with an impaired fibrinolytic activity and elevated plasminogen activator inhibitor-1. Metabolism. 1990;39(10):1044-1048.

91. Alessi M-C, Juhan-Vague I. PAI-1 and the Metabolic Syndrome. Arteriosclerosis, Thrombosis, and Vascular Biology. October 1, 2006 2006;26(10):2200-2207.

92. Mertens I, Verrijken A, Michiels JJ, Van der Planken M, Ruige JB, Van Gaal LF. Among inflammation and coagulation markers, PAI-1 is a true component of the metabolic syndrome. Int J Obes. 2006;30(8):1308-1314.

93. Kuo HK, Yen CJ, Chang CH, Kuo CK, Chen JH, Sorond F. Relation of C-reactive protein to stroke, cognitive disorders, and depression in the general population: systematic review and meta-analysis. Lancet neurology. Jun 2005;4(6):371-380.

94. Pierce BL, Ballard-Barbash R, Bernstein L, et al. Elevated Biomarkers of Inflammation Are Associated With Reduced Survival Among Breast Cancer Patients. Journal of Clinical Oncology. July 20, 2009 2009;27(21):3437-3444.

95. Forsythe C, Phinney S, Feinman R, et al. Limited Effect of Dietary Saturated Fat on Plasma Saturated Fat in the Context of a Low Carbohydrate Diet. Lipids. 2010;45(10):947-962.

96. Forsythe C, Phinney S, Fernandez M, et al. Comparison of Low Fat and Low Carbohydrate Diets on Circulating Fatty Acid Composition and Markers of Inflammation. Lipids. 2008;43(1):65-77.

97. Volek J, Phinney S, Forsythe C, et al. Carbohydrate Restriction has a More Favorable Impact on the Metabolic Syndrome than a Low Fat Diet. Lipids. 2009;44(4):297-309.

98. Hession M, Rolland C, Kulkarni U, Wise A, Broom J. Systematic review of randomized controlled trials of low-carbohydrate vs. low-fat/low-calorie diets in the management of obesity and its comorbidities. Obesity Reviews. 2009;10(1):36-50.

99. Anderson JJ, Rondano P, Holmes A. Roles of diet and physical activity in the prevention of osteoporosis. Scandinavian journal of rheumatology. Supplement. 1996;103:65-74.

100. Trapp EG, Chisholm DJ, Freund J, Boutcher SH. The effects of high-intensity intermittent exercise training on fat loss and fasting insulin levels of young women. International Journal of Obesity. 2008;32(4):684-691.

101. Bray GA, Smith SR, de Jonge L, et al. Effect of Dietary Protein Content on Weight Gain, Energy Expenditure, and Body Composition During Overeating. JAMA: The Journal of the American Medical Association. January 4, 2012 2012;307(1):47-55.

102. Andersson A, Tengblad S, Karlström B, et al. Whole-Grain Foods Do Not Affect Insulin Sensitivity or Markers of Lipid Peroxidation and Inflammation in Healthy, Moderately Overweight Subjects. The Journal of nutrition. June 1, 2007 2007;137(6):1401-1407.

103. Singh M, Krikorian AD. Inhibition of trypsin activity in vitro by phytate. Journal of agricultural and food chemistry. 1982/07/01 1982;30(4):799-800.

104. Burkholder J, Libra B, Weyer P, et al. Impacts of waste from concentrated animal feeding operations on water quality. Environmental health perspectives. Feb 2007;115(2):308-312.

105. Cordain L, Toohey L, Smith MJ, Hickey MS. Modulation of immune function by dietary lectins in rheumatoid arthritis. The British journal of nutrition. Mar 2000;83(3):207-217.

106. Miyake K, Tanaka T, McNeil PL. Lectin-based food poisoning: a new mechanism of protein toxicity. PloS one. 2007;2(8):e687.

107. Freed DL. Do dietary lectins cause disease? BMJ. Apr 17 1999;318(7190):1023-1024.

108. Jonsson T, Olsson S, Ahren B, Bog-Hansen TC, Dole A, Lindeberg S. Agrarian diet and diseases of affluence--do evolutionary novel dietary lectins cause leptin resistance? BMC endocrine disorders. 2005;5:10.

109. Ciardiello F, Tortora G. EGFR Antagonists in Cancer Treatment. New England Journal of Medicine. 2008;358(11):1160-1174.

110. Rubin R, Baserga R. Insulin-like growth factor-I receptor. Its role in cell proliferation, apoptosis, and tumorigenicity. Laboratory investigation; a journal of technical methods and pathology. Sep 1995;73(3):311-331.

111. Kilpatrick DC. Mechanisms and assessment of lectin-mediated mitogenesis. Molecular biotechnology. Feb 1999;11(1):55-65.

112. Frazer AC, Fletcher RF, Ross CA, Shaw B, Sammons HG, Schneider R. Gluten-induced enteropathy: the effect of partially digested gluten. Lancet. 1959;2(7097):252-255.
113. Bodinier M, Legoux MA, Pineau F, et al. Intestinal translocation capabilities of wheat allergens using the Caco-2 cell line. Journal of agricultural and food chemistry. May 30 2007;55(11):4576-4583.
114. Thomas KE, Sapone A, Fasano A, Vogel SN. Gliadin stimulation of murine macrophage inflammatory gene expression and intestinal permeability are MyD88-dependent: role of the innate immune response in Celiac disease. Journal of immunology. Feb 15 2006;176(4):2512-2521.
115. Detlef S. Current Concepts of Celiac Disease Pathogenesis. Gastroenterology. 2000;119(1):234-242.
116. Fasano A. Systemic autoimmune disorders in celiac disease. Current Opinion in Gastroenterology. 2006;22(6):674-679 610.1097/1001.mog.0000245543.00 00272537.0000245549e.
117. Wahab PJ, Crusius JB, Meijer JW, Mulder CJ. Gluten challenge in borderline gluten-sensitive enteropathy. The American journal of gastroenterology. May 2001;96(5):1464-1469.
118. Hadjivassiliou M, Grünewald RA, Chattopadhyay AK, et al. Clinical, radiological, neurophysiological, and neuropathological characteristics of gluten ataxia. The Lancet. 1998;352(9140):1582-1585.
119. Hernandez-Lahoz C, Mauri-Capdevila G, Vega-Villar J, Rodrigo L. [Neurological disorders associated with gluten sensitivity]. Revista de neurologia. Sep 1 2011;53(5):287-300.
120. Briani C, Zara G, Alaedini A, et al. Neurological complications of celiac disease and autoimmune mechanisms: a prospective study. Journal of neuroimmunology. Mar 2008;195(1-2):171-175.

121. Singh M, Kay. Wheat gluten as a pathogenic factor in schizophrenia. Science. January 30, 1976 1976;191(4225):401-402.

122. Fry L, Riches DJ, Seah PP, Hoffbrand AV. Clearance of Skin Leasion in Dermatitis Herpetiformis After Gluten Withdrawal. The Lancet. 1973;301(7798):288-291.

123. Workman EM, Alun Jones V, Wilson AJ, Hunter JO. Diet in the management of Crohn's disease. Human nutrition. Applied nutrition. Dec 1984;38(6):469-473.

124. Knivsberg AM, Reichelt KL, Hoien T, Nodland M. A randomised, controlled study of dietary intervention in autistic syndromes. Nutritional neuroscience. Sep 2002;5(4):251-261.

125. King M, Bearman P. Diagnostic change and the increased prevalence of autism. International Journal of Epidemiology. October 1, 2009 2009;38(5):1224-1234.

126. Millward C, Ferriter M, Calver S, Connell-Jones G. Gluten- and casein-free diets for autistic spectrum disorder. Cochrane database of systematic reviews. 2004(2):CD003498.

127. De Santis A, Addolorato G, Romito A, et al. Schizophrenic symptoms and SPECT abnormalities in a coeliac patient: regression after a gluten-free diet. Journal of internal medicine. Nov 1997;242(5):421-423.

128. Stazi AV, Trinti B. Selenium status and over-expression of interleukin-15 in celiac disease and autoimmune thyroid diseases. Annali dell'Istituto Superiore di Sanità. 2010;46:389-399.

129. Price KR, Johnson IT, Fenwick GR. The chemistry and biological significance of saponins in foods and feeding-stuffs. Critical reviews in food science and nutrition. 1987;26(1):27-135.

130. Johnson IT, Gee JM, Price K, Curl C, Fenwick GR. Influence of saponins on gut permeability and active nutrient transport in vitro. The Journal of nutrition. Nov

1986;116(11):2270-2277.

131. Warren HS, Fitting C, Hoff E, et al. Resilience to Bacterial Infection: Difference between Species Could Be Due to Proteins in Serum. Journal of Infectious Diseases. January 15, 2010 2010;201(2):223-232.

132. Khafipour E, Krause DO, Plaizier JC. A grain-based subacute ruminal acidosis challenge causes translocation of lipopolysaccharide and triggers inflammation. Journal of Dairy Science. 2009;92(3):1060-1070.

133. Jenkins DJA, Kendall CWC, Augustin LSA, et al. Effect of Wheat Bran on Glycemic Control and Risk Factors for Cardiovascular Disease in Type 2 Diabetes. Diabetes Care. September 1, 2002 2002;25(9):1522-1528.

134. Stender S, Dyerberg J, Astrup A. High Levels of Industrially Produced Trans Fat in Popular Fast Foods. New England Journal of Medicine. 2006;354(15):1650-1652.

135. De Roos NM, Schouten EG, Scheek LM, van Tol A, Katan MB. Replacement of dietary saturated fat with trans fat reduces serum paraoxonase activity in healthy men and women. Metabolism: clinical and experimental. 2002;51(12):1534-1537.

136. Lopez-Garcia E, Schulze MB, Meigs JB, et al. Consumption of Trans Fatty Acids Is Related to Plasma Biomarkers of Inflammation and Endothelial Dysfunction. The Journal of nutrition. March 1, 2005 2005;135(3):562-566.

137. Kritchevsky D. Diet and cancer. CA: A Cancer Journal for Clinicians. 1991;41(6):328-333.

138. Carroll K. Dietary fats and cancer. The American journal of clinical nutrition. April 1, 1991 1991;53(4):1064S-1067S.

139. Lee Pearce M, Dayton S. Incidence of Cancer in Men on a Diet High in Polyunsaturated Fat. The Lancet. 1971;297(7697):464-467.

140. Wyatt D. Simultaneous analysis of BHA, TBHQ, BHT and propyl gallate by gas chromatography as extracted

from refined vegetable oil. Journal of the American Oil Chemists' Society. 1981;58(10):917-920.

141. Ito N, Fukushima S, Tsuda H. Carcinogenicity and Modification of the Carcinogenic Response by bha, Bht, and Other Antioxidants. Critical Reviews in Toxicology. 1985;15(2):109-150.

142. Quinn L, Tang H. Antioxidant properties of phenolic compounds in macadamia nuts. Journal of the American Oil Chemists' Society. 1996;73(11):1585-1588.

143. Marisa M W. Functional lipid characteristics, oxidative stability, and antioxidant activity of macadamia nut (Macadamia integrifolia) cultivars. Food Chemistry. 2010;121(4):1103-1108.

144. Kritchevsky D. Antimutagenic and some other effects of conjugated linoleic acid. The British journal of nutrition. May 2000;83(5):459-465.

145. Chin SF, Liu W, Storkson JM, Ha YL, Pariza MW. Dietary sources of conjugated dienoic isomers of linoleic acid, a newly recognized class of anticarcinogens. Journal of Food Composition and Analysis. 1992;5(3):185-197.

146. Dhiman TR, Anand GR, Satter LD, Pariza MW. Conjugated Linoleic Acid Content of Milk from Cows Fed Different Diets1. Journal of dairy science. 1999;82(10):2146-2156.

147. Pariza MW, Ashoor SH, Chu FS, Lund DB. Effects of temperature and time on mutagen formation in pan-fried hamburger. Cancer Letters. 1979;7(2-3):63-69.

148. Champ CE, Mishra MV, Showalter TN, Ohri N, Dicker AP, Simone NL. Dietary Recommendations During and After Cancer Treatment: Consistently Inconsistent? Nutrition and cancer. April 1, 2013 2013;65(3):430-439.

149. Ip C, Chin SF, Scimeca JA, Pariza MW. Mammary Cancer Prevention by Conjugated Dienoic Derivative of Linoleic Acid. Cancer research. November 15, 1991 1991;51(22):6118-6124.

150. Cesano A, Visonneau S, Scimeca JA, Kritchevsky D, Santoli D. Opposite effects of linoleic acid and conjugated linoleic acid on human prostatic cancer in SCID mice. Anticancer research. 1998;18(3A):1429-1434.

151. Ha YL, Storkson J, Pariza MW. Inhibition of Benzo(a) pyrene-induced Mouse Forestomach Neoplasia by Conjugated Dienoic Derivatives of Linoleic Acid. Cancer research. February 15, 1990 1990;50(4):1097-1101.

152. Nutter M, Lockhart E, Harris R. The chemical composition of depot fats in chickens and turkeys. Journal of the American Oil Chemists' Society. 1943;20(11):231-234.

153. Welsch CW. Relationship between Dietary Fat and Experimental Mammary Tumorigenesis: A Review and Critique. Cancer research. April 1, 1992 1992;52(7 Supplement):2040s-2048s.

154. Aro A, Mannisto S, Salminen I, Ovaskainen ML, Kataja V, Uusitupa M. Inverse association between dietary and serum conjugated linoleic acid and risk of breast cancer in postmenopausal women. Nutrition and cancer. 2000;38(2):151-157.

155. Rakoff-Nahoum S. Why cancer and inflammation? The Yale journal of biology and medicine. Dec 2006;79(3-4):123-130.

156. Kritchevsky D, Tepper S, Wright S, Czarnecki S, Wilson T, Nicolosi R. Conjugated linoleic acid isomer effects in atherosclerosis: Growth and regression of lesions. Lipids. 2004;39(7):611-616.

157. Brown JM, McIntosh MK. Conjugated Linoleic Acid in Humans: Regulation of Adiposity and Insulin Sensitivity. The Journal of nutrition. October 1, 2003 2003;133(10):3041-3046.

158. Smedman A, Vessby B. Conjugated linoleic acid supplementation in humans--metabolic effects. Lipids. Aug 2001;36(8):773-781.

159. Ip C, Scimeca JA, Thompson H. Effect of timing and

duration of dietary conjugated linoleic acid on mammary cancer prevention. Nutrition and cancer. 1995/01/01 1995;24(3):241-247.

160. Ha YL, Grimm NK, Pariza MW. Newly recognized anticarcinogenic fatty acids: identification and quantification in natural and processed cheeses. Journal of agricultural and food chemistry. 1989/01/01 1989;37(1):75-81.

161. Ritzenthaler KL, McGuire MK, Falen R, Shultz TD, Dasgupta N, McGuire MA. Estimation of Conjugated Linoleic Acid Intake by Written Dietary Assessment Methodologies Underestimates Actual Intake Evaluated by Food Duplicate Methodology. The Journal of nutrition. May 1, 2001 2001;131(5):1548-1554.

162. Kelley NS, Hubbard NE, Erickson KL. Conjugated Linoleic Acid Isomers and Cancer. The Journal of nutrition. December 1, 2007 2007;137(12):2599-2607.

163. Brown JM, Halvorsen YD, Lea-Currie YR, Geigerman C, McIntosh M. Trans-10, Cis-12, But Not Cis-9, Trans-11, Conjugated Linoleic Acid Attenuates Lipogenesis in Primary Cultures of Stromal Vascular Cells from Human Adipose Tissue. The Journal of nutrition. September 1, 2001 2001;131(9):2316-2321.

164. Cho HJ, Kim EJ, Lim SS, et al. Trans-10,cis-12, Not cis-9,trans-11, Conjugated Linoleic Acid Inhibits G1-S Progression in HT-29 Human Colon Cancer Cells. The Journal of nutrition. April 1, 2006 2006;136(4):893-898.

165. Veierød MB, Laake P, Thelle DS. Dietary fat intake and risk of prostate cancer: A prospective study of 25,708 Norwegian men. International Journal of Cancer. 1997;73(5):634-638.

166. Daley C, Abbott A, Doyle P, Nader G, Larson S. A review of fatty acid profiles and antioxidant content in grass-fed and grain-fed beef. Nutrition Journal. 2010;9(1):10.

167. Simopoulos AP. Essential fatty acids in health and chronic disease. The American Journal of Clinical Nutrition.

September 1, 1999 1999;70(3):560S-569S.

168. Vedin I, Cederholm T, Freund Levi Y, et al. Effects of docosahexaenoic acid-rich n-3 fatty acid supplementation on cytokine release from blood mononuclear leukocytes: the OmegAD study. The American journal of clinical nutrition. June 1, 2008 2008;87(6):1616-1622.

169. Norrish AE, Skeaff CM, Arribas GL, Sharpe SJ, Jackson RT. Prostate cancer risk and consumption of fish oils: a dietary biomarker-based case-control study. Br J Cancer. 1999;81(7):1238-1242.

170. Terry P, Lichtenstein P, Feychting M, Ahlbom A, Wolk A. Fatty fish consumption and risk of prostate cancer. Lancet. 2001;357(9270):1764-1766.

171. Greene ER, Huang S, Serhan CN, Panigrahy D. Regulation of inflammation in cancer by eicosanoids. Prostaglandins & other lipid mediators. Nov 2011;96(1-4):27-36.

172. Simopoulos AP. Omega-3 Fatty Acids in Inflammation and Autoimmune Diseases. Journal of the American College of Nutrition. December 1, 2002 2002;21(6):495-505.

173. Williams CD, Whitley BM, Hoyo C, et al. A high ratio of dietary n-6/n-3 polyunsaturated fatty acids is associated with increased risk of prostate cancer. Nutrition research. Jan 2011;31(1):1-8.

174. Nuernberg K, Nuernberg G, Ender K, et al. N-3 fatty acids and conjugated linoleic acids of longissimus muscle in beef cattle. European Journal of Lipid Science and Technology. 2002;104(8):463-471.

175. van Vliet T, Katan MB. Lower ratio of n-3 to n-6 fatty acids in cultured than in wild fish. The American Journal of Clinical Nutrition. Jan 1990;51(1):1-2.

176. Simopoulos AP, Salem N, Jr. n-3 fatty acids in eggs from range-fed Greek chickens. The New England journal of medicine. Nov 16 1989;321(20):1412.

177. Sun H, Hu Y, Gu Z, Owens RT, Chen YQ, Edwards IJ.

Omega-3 fatty acids induce apoptosis in human breast cancer cells and mouse mammary tissue through syndecan-1 inhibition of the MEK-Erk pathway. Carcinogenesis. Oct 2011;32(10):1518-1524.

178. Cockbain AJ, Toogood GJ, Hull MA. Omega-3 polyunsaturated fatty acids for the treatment and prevention of colorectal cancer. Gut. Jan 2012;61(1):135-149.

179. Friedrichs W, Ruparel SB, Marciniak RA, deGraffenried L. Omega-3 fatty acid inhibition of prostate cancer progression to hormone independence is associated with suppression of mTOR signaling and androgen receptor expression. Nutrition and cancer. 2011;63(5):771-777.

180. Bougnoux P, Germain E, Chajes V, et al. Cytotoxic drugs efficacy correlates with adipose tissue docosahexaenoic acid level in locally advanced breast carcinoma. Br J Cancer. Apr 1999;79(11-12):1765-1769.

181. Feng Z, Hu W, Hu Y, Tang MS. Acrolein is a major cigarette-related lung cancer agent: Preferential binding at p53 mutational hotspots and inhibition of DNA repair. Proc Natl Acad Sci U S A. Oct 17 2006;103(42):15404-15409.

182. Tang MS, Wang HT, Hu Y, et al. Acrolein induced DNA damage, mutagenicity and effect on DNA repair. Molecular nutrition & food research. Sep 2011;55(9):1291-1300.

183. Wu S-C, Yen G-C. Effects of cooking oil fumes on the genotoxicity and oxidative stress in human lung carcinoma (A-549) cells. Toxicology in Vitro. 2004;18(5):571-580.

184. Qu YH, Xu GX, Zhou JZ, et al. Genotoxicity of heated cooking oil vapors. Mutation Research/Genetic Toxicology. 1992;298(2):105-111.

185. Lam WK. Lung cancer in Asian women-the environment and genes. Respirology. Sep 2005;10(4):408-417.

186. Hosgood HD, 3rd, Berndt SI, Lan Q. GST genotypes and lung cancer susceptibility in Asian populations with

indoor air pollution exposures: a meta-analysis. Mutation research. Nov-Dec 2007;636(1-3):134-143.

187. Takeuchi K, Kato M, Suzuki H, et al. Acrolein induces activation of the epidermal growth factor receptor of human keratinocytes for cell death. Journal of cellular biochemistry. 2001;81(4):679-688.

188. Grootveld M, Silwood CJL, Addis P, Claxson A, Serra BB, Viana M. Health Effects of Oxidized Heated Oils. Foodservice Research International. 2001;13(1):41-55.

189. Esterbauer H. Cytotoxicity and genotoxicity of lipid-oxidation products. The American journal of clinical nutrition. May 1993;57(5 Suppl):779S-785S; discussion 785S-786S.

190. Staprans I, Rapp J, Pan X, Kim K, Feingold K. Oxidized lipids in the diet are a source of oxidized lipid in chylomicrons of human serum. Arteriosclerosis, Thrombosis, and Vascular Biology. December 1, 1994 1994;14(12):1900-1905.

191. Chong YH, Ng TK. Effects of palm oil on cardiovascular risk. The Medical journal of Malaysia. Mar 1991;46(1):41-50.

192. Ebong PE, Owu DU, Isong EU. Influence of palm oil (Elaesis guineensis) on health. Plant Foods for Human Nutrition (Formerly Qualitas Plantarum). 1999;53(3):209-222.

193. Kanner J, Lapidot T. The stomach as a bioreactor: dietary lipid peroxidation in the gastric fluid and the effects of plant-derived antioxidants. Free Radical Biology and Medicine. 2001;31(11):1388-1395.

194. Yoshida H. Influence of fatty acids of different unsaturation in the oxidation of purified vegetable oils during microwave irradiation. Journal of the Science of Food and Agriculture. 1993;62(1):41-47.

195. Felton CV, Crook D, Davies MJ, Oliver MF. Dietary polyunsaturated fatty acids and composition of human

aortic plaques. Lancet. Oct 29 1994;344(8931):1195-
1196.

196. Ibrahim A, Natrajan S, Ghafoorunissa R. Dietary
trans-fatty acids alter adipocyte plasma membrane fatty
acid composition and insulin sensitivity in rats. Metabolism: clinical and experimental. Feb 2005;54(2):240-246.

197. Lemaitre RN, King IB, Raghunathan TE, et al. Cell Membrane Trans-Fatty Acids and the Risk of Primary Cardiac
Arrest. Circulation. February 12, 2002 2002;105(6):697-
701.

198. Wahls TL. Telling the World. Ann Intern Med. July 1,
2008 2008;149(1):61-62.

199. Wahls T. The Seventy Percent Solution. Journal of General Internal Medicine. 2011;26(10):1215-1216.

200. O'Keefe Jr JH, Cordain L. Cardiovascular Disease Resulting From a Diet and Lifestyle at Odds With Our Paleolithic Genome: How to Become a 21st-Century Hunter-Gatherer. Mayo Clinic Proceedings. 2004;79(1):101-108.

201. Eaton SB, Eaton SB, 3rd, Konner MJ. Paleolithic nutrition revisited: a twelve-year retrospective on its nature
and implications. Eur J Clin Nutr. Apr 1997;51(4):207-
216.

202. Cordain L, Eaton SB, Sebastian A, et al. Origins and
evolution of the Western diet: health implications for
the 21st century. The American Journal of Clinical Nutrition. February 1, 2005 2005;81(2):341-354.

203. Grotto D, Zied E. The Standard American Diet and
Its Relationship to the Health Status of Americans.
Nutrition in Clinical Practice. December 1, 2010
2010;25(6):603-612.

204. MRC/BHF Heart Protection Study of antioxidant vitamin supplementation in 20,536 high-risk individuals: a randomised placebo-controlled trial. Lancet. Jul 6
2002;360(9326):23-33.

205. Cook NR, Albert CM, Gaziano JM, et al. A random-

ized factorial trial of vitamins C and E and beta carotene in the secondary prevention of cardiovascular events in women: results from the Women's Antioxidant Cardiovascular Study. Archives of internal medicine. Aug 13-27 2007;167(15):1610-1618.

206. Albert CM, Cook NR, Gaziano JM, et al. Effect of folic acid and B vitamins on risk of cardiovascular events and total mortality among women at high risk for cardiovascular disease: a randomized trial. Jama. May 7 2008;299(17):2027-2036.

207. Zhang SM, Cook NR, Albert CM, Gaziano JM, Buring JE, Manson JE. Effect of combined folic acid, vitamin B6, and vitamin B12 on cancer risk in women: a randomized trial. Jama. Nov 5 2008;300(17):2012-2021.

208. Joshipura KJ, Hu FB, Manson JE, et al. The Effect of Fruit and Vegetable Intake on Risk for Coronary Heart Disease. Ann Intern Med. June 19, 2001 2001;134(12):1106-1114.

209. Dietary supplementation with n-3 polyunsaturated fatty acids and vitamin E after myocardial infarction: results of the GISSI-Prevenzione trial. Gruppo Italiano per lo Studio della Sopravvivenza nell'Infarto miocardico. Lancet. Aug 7 1999;354(9177):447-455.

210. Lippman SM, Klein EA, Goodman PJ, et al. Effect of Selenium and Vitamin E on Risk of Prostate Cancer and Other Cancers. JAMA: The Journal of the American Medical Association. January 7, 2009 2009;301(1):39-51.

211. Ebbing M, Bonaa KH, Nygard O, et al. Cancer incidence and mortality after treatment with folic acid and vitamin B12. Jama. Nov 18 2009;302(19):2119-2126.

212. Ulrich CM, Potter JD. Folate Supplementation: Too Much of a Good Thing? Cancer Epidemiology Biomarkers & Prevention. February 1, 2006 2006;15(2):189-193.

213. Bjelakovic G, Gluud LL, Nikolova D, et al. Vitamin D supplementation for prevention of mortality

in adults. Cochrane database of systematic reviews. 2011(7):CD007470.

214. Houghton LA, Vieth R. The case against ergocalciferol (vitamin D2) as a vitamin supplement. The American journal of clinical nutrition. Oct 2006;84(4):694-697.

215. Williamson CS, Foster RK, Stanner SA, Buttriss JL. Red meat in the diet. Nutrition Bulletin. 2005;30(4):323-355.

216. Pauletto P, Puato M, Caroli MG, et al. Blood pressure and atherogenic lipoprotein profiles of fish-diet and vegetarian villagers in Tanzania: The Lugalawa study. Lancet. 1996;348(9030):784-788.

217. Bang HO, Dyerberg J, Nielsen AB. Plasma lipid and lipoprotein pattern in Greenlandic West-coast Eskimos. Lancet. 1971;1(7710):1143-1145.

218. Patel AM, Goldfarb S. Got calcium? Welcome to the calcium-alkali syndrome. Journal of the American Society of Nephrology : JASN. Sep 2010;21(9):1440-1443.

219. Paspati I, Galanos A, Lyritis GP. Hip fracture epidemiology in Greece during 1977-1992. Calcified tissue international. Jun 1998;62(6):542-547.

220. Weaver CM, Heaney RP, Martin BR, Fitzsimmons ML. Human calcium absorption from whole-wheat products. The Journal of nutrition. Nov 1991;121(11):1769-1775.

221. Lonnerdal B, Sandberg AS, Sandstrom B, Kunz C. Inhibitory effects of phytic acid and other inositol phosphates on zinc and calcium absorption in suckling rats. The Journal of nutrition. 1989;119(2):211-214.

222. Heaney RP, Dowell MS, Hale CA, Bendich A. Calcium Absorption Varies within the Reference Range for Serum 25-Hydroxyvitamin D. Journal of the American College of Nutrition. April 1, 2003 2003;22(2):142-146.

223. Ulitsky A, Ananthakrishnan AN, Naik A, et al. Vitamin D Deficiency in Patients With Inflammatory Bowel Disease. Journal of Parenteral and Enteral Nutrition. May 1, 2011 2011;35(3):308-316.

224. Basha B, Rao DS, Han ZH, Parfitt AM. Osteomalacia due to vitamin D depletion: a neglected consequence of intestinal malabsorption. The American journal of medicine. Mar 2000;108(4):296-300.

225. Kamao M, Suhara Y, Tsugawa N, et al. Vitamin K content of foods and dietary vitamin K intake in Japanese young women. Journal of nutritional science and vitaminology. Dec 2007;53(6):464-470.

226. Elder SJ, Haytowitz DB, Howe J, Peterson JW, Booth SL. Vitamin k contents of meat, dairy, and fast food in the u.s. Diet. Journal of agricultural and food chemistry. Jan 25 2006;54(2):463-467.

227. Hannan MT, Tucker KL, Dawson-Hughes B, Cupples LA, Felson DT, Kiel DP. Effect of dietary protein on bone loss in elderly men and women: the Framingham Osteoporosis Study. Journal of bone and mineral research : the official journal of the American Society for Bone and Mineral Research. Dec 2000;15(12):2504-2512.

228. Schurch M-A, Rizzoli R, Slosman D, Vadas L, Vergnaud P, Bonjour J-P. Protein Supplements Increase Serum Insulin-Like Growth Factor-I Levels and Attenuate Proximal Femur Bone Loss in Patients with Recent Hip Fracture. Annals of internal medicine. May 15, 1998 1998;128(10):801-809.

229. Kerstetter JE, Looker AC, Insogna KL. Low dietary protein and low bone density. Calcified tissue international. Apr 2000;66(4):313.

230. Suominen H. Muscle training for bone strength. Aging clinical and experimental research. Apr 2006;18(2):85-93.

231. Wilks DC, Winwood K, Gilliver SF, et al. Bone mass and geometry of the tibia and the radius of master sprinters, middle and long distance runners, race-walkers and sedentary control participants: a pQCT study. Bone. Jul 2009;45(1):91-97.

232. Layne JE, Nelson ME. The effects of progressive resistance training on bone density: a review. Medicine and science in sports and exercise. Jan 1999;31(1):25-30.

233. Bischoff-Ferrari HA, Kiel DP, Dawson-Hughes B, et al. Dietary calcium and serum 25-hydroxyvitamin D status in relation to BMD among U.S. adults. Journal of bone and mineral research : the official journal of the American Society for Bone and Mineral Research. May 2009;24(5):935-942.

234. DeFronzo RA, Cooke CR, Andres R, Faloona GR, Davis PJ. The effect of insulin on renal handling of sodium, potassium, calcium, and phosphate in man. The Journal of clinical investigation. Apr 1975;55(4):845-855.

235. Holl MG, Allen LH. Sucrose ingestion, insulin response and mineral metabolism in humans. The Journal of nutrition. Jul 1987;117(7):1229-1233.

236. Bolland MJ, Barber PA, Doughty RN, et al. Vascular events in healthy older women receiving calcium supplementation: randomised controlled trial. BMJ. 2008-01-31 23:01:24 2008;336(7638):262-266.

237. Xiao Q, Murphy RA, Houston DK, Harris TB, Chow W, Park Y. Dietary and supplemental calcium intake and cardiovascular disease mortality: The national institutes of health–aarp diet and health study. JAMA Internal Medicine. 2013;173(8):639-646.

238. Li K, Kaaks R, Linseisen J, Rohrmann S. Associations of dietary calcium intake and calcium supplementation with myocardial infarction and stroke risk and overall cardiovascular mortality in the Heidelberg cohort of the European Prospective Investigation into Cancer and Nutrition study (EPIC-Heidelberg). Heart. June 15, 2012 2012;98(12):920-925.

239. Van Hemelrijck M, Michaelsson K, Linseisen J, Rohrmann S. Calcium Intake and Serum Concentration in Relation to Risk of Cardiovascular Death in NHANES

III. PLoS ONE. 2013;8(4):e61037.

240. Schurgers LJ, Spronk HMH, Soute BAM, Schiffers PM, DeMey JGR, Vermeer C. Regression of warfarin-induced medial elastocalcinosis by high intake of vitamin K in rats. Blood. April 1, 2007 2007;109(7):2823-2831.

241. Breslau NA. Calcium, estrogen, and progestin in the treatment of osteoporosis. Rheumatic diseases clinics of North America. Aug 1994;20(3):691-716.

242. Grady D, Gebretsadik T, Kerlikowske K, Ernster V, Petitti D. Hormone replacement therapy and endometrial cancer risk: A meta-analysis. Obstetrics & Gynecology. 1995;85(2):304-313.

243. Schairer C, Lubin J, Troisi R, Sturgeon S, Brinton L, Hoover R. Menopausal Estrogen and Estrogen-Progestin Replacement Therapy and Breast Cancer Risk. JAMA: The Journal of the American Medical Association. January 26, 2000 2000;283(4):485-491.

244. Black DM, Delmas PD, Eastell R, et al. Once-yearly zoledronic acid for treatment of postmenopausal osteoporosis. The New England journal of medicine. May 3 2007;356(18):1809-1822.

245. Chesnut CH, 3rd, McClung MR, Ensrud KE, et al. Alendronate treatment of the postmenopausal osteoporotic woman: effect of multiple dosages on bone mass and bone remodeling. The American journal of medicine. Aug 1995;99(2):144-152.

246. Morris JN, Chave SPW, Adam C, Sirey C, Epstein L, Sheehan DJ. Vigorous Exercise in Leisure-Time and the Incidence of Coronary Heart-Disease. The Lancet. 1973;301(7799):333-339.

247. Thompson HJ. Effect of Exercise Intensity and Duration on the Induction of Mammary Carcinogenesis. Cancer Research. April 1, 1994 1994;54(7 Supplement):1960s-1963s.

248. Morris JN, Pollard R, Everitt MG, Chave SPW, Sem-

mence AM. Vigorous Exercise in Leisure-Time and the Incidence of Coronary Heart-Disease. The Lancet. 1980;316(8206):1207-1210.

249. Kokkinos P, Myers J, Faselis C, et al. Exercise Capacity and Mortality in Older Men. Circulation. August 24, 2010 2010;122(8):790-797.

250. Kokkinos P, Myers J, Kokkinos JP, et al. Exercise Capacity and Mortality in Black and White Men. Circulation. February 5, 2008 2008;117(5):614-622.

251. O'Keefe JH, Vogel R, Lavie CJ, Cordain L. Exercise Like a Hunter-Gatherer: A Prescription for Organic Physical Fitness. Progress in Cardiovascular Diseases. 2011;53(6):471-479.

252. Nader Pr BRHHRMMSLOBM. Moderate-to-vigorous physical activity from ages 9 to 15 years. JAMA: The Journal of the American Medical Association. 2008;300(3):295-305.

253. Perrier-Great Waters of France I. The Perrier study: Fitness in America. New York: Perrier-Great Waters of France, Inc.; 1979.

254. Hill K, Kaplan H, Hawkes K, Hurtado A. Men's time allocation to subsistence work among the Ache of Eastern Paraguay. Human Ecology. 1985;13(1):29-47.

255. Walker R, Hill K. Modeling growth and senescence in physical performance among the ache of eastern paraguay. American Journal of Human Biology. 2003;15(2):196-208.

256. Mbalilaki JA, Masesa Z, Stromme SB, et al. Daily energy expenditure and cardiovascular risk in Masai, rural and urban Bantu Tanzanians. British journal of sports medicine. Feb 2010;44(2):121-126.

257. La Gerche A, Burns AT, Mooney DJ, et al. Exercise-induced right ventricular dysfunction and structural remodelling in endurance athletes. European Heart Journal. December 6, 2011 2011.

258. Neilan TG, Januzzi JL, Lee-Lewandrowski E, et al. Myocardial Injury and Ventricular Dysfunction Related to Training Levels Among Nonelite Participants in the Boston Marathon. Circulation. November 28, 2006 2006;114(22):2325-2333.

259. Banks L, Sasson Z, Esfandiari S, Busato G-M, Goodman JM. Cardiac function following prolonged exercise: influence of age. Journal of Applied Physiology. June 1, 2011 2011;110(6):1541-1548.

260. Nottin S, Doucende G, Schuster I, Tanguy S, Dauzat M, Obert P. Alteration in Left Ventricular Strains and Torsional Mechanics After Ultralong Duration Exercise in Athletes/Clinical Perspective. Circulation: Cardiovascular Imaging. July 1, 2009 2009;2(4):323-330.

261. Pelliccia A, Kinoshita N, Pisicchio C, et al. Long-Term Clinical Consequences of Intense, Uninterrupted Endurance Training in Olympic Athletes. J Am Coll Cardiol. April 13, 2010 2010;55(15):1619-1625.

262. Wilson M, O'Hanlon R, Prasad S, et al. Diverse patterns of myocardial fibrosis in lifelong, veteran endurance athletes. Journal of Applied Physiology. Jun 2011;110(6):1622-1626.

263. Trivax JE, Franklin BA, Goldstein JA, et al. Acute cardiac effects of marathon running. Journal of Applied Physiology. May 1, 2010 2010;108(5):1148-1153.

264. Urhausen A, Gabriel H, Kindermann W. Blood hormones as markers of training stress and overtraining. Sports medicine (Auckland, N.Z.). 1995;20(4):251-276.

265. Kim JH, Malhotra R, Chiampas G, et al. Cardiac Arrest during Long-Distance Running Races. New England Journal of Medicine. 2012;366(2):130-140.

266. Hootman JM, Macera CA, Ainsworth BE, Martin M, Addy CL, Blair SN. Association among Physical Activity Level, Cardiorespiratory Fitness, and Risk of Musculoskeletal Injury. American journal of epidemiology. Au-

gust 1, 2001 2001;154(3):251-258.

267. Koplan JP, Siscovick DS, Goldbaum GM. The risks of exercise: a public health view of injuries and hazards. Public health reports. Mar-Apr 1985;100(2):189-195.

268. Lysholm J, Wiklander J. Injuries in runners. The American Journal of Sports Medicine. March 1987 1987;15(2):168-171.

269. Burgomaster KA, Heigenhauser GJF, Gibala MJ. Effect of short-term sprint interval training on human skeletal muscle carbohydrate metabolism during exercise and time-trial performance. Journal of Applied Physiology. 2006;100(6):2041-2047.

270. Burgomaster KA, Howarth KR, Phillips SM, et al. Similar metabolic adaptations during exercise after low volume sprint interval and traditional endurance training in humans. Journal of Physiology. 2008;586(1):151-160.

271. Sandvei M, Jeppesen PB, Stoen L, et al. Sprint interval running increases insulin sensitivity in young healthy subjects. Archives of Physiology and Biochemistry. 2012;118(3):139-147.

272. Ristow M, Schmeisser S. Extending life span by increasing oxidative stress. Free Radical Biology and Medicine. 2011;51(2):327-336.

273. Schulz TJ, Zarse K, Voigt A, Urban N, Birringer M, Ristow M. Glucose restriction extends Caenorhabditis elegans life span by inducing mitochondrial respiration and increasing oxidative stress. Cell metabolism. Oct 2007;6(4):280-293.

274. Criswell D, Powers S, Dodd S, et al. High intensity training-induced changes in skeletal muscle antioxidant enzyme activity. Medicine and science in sports and exercise. 1993;25(10):1135-1140.

275. Little JP, Safdar A, Wilkin GP, Tarnopolsky MA, Gibala MJ. A practical model of low-volume high-intensity interval training induces mitochondrial biogenesis in human skeletal muscle: potential mechanisms. The Journal of Physiology. March 15, 2010 2010;588(6):1011-1022.

276. Haigis MC, Guarente LP. Mammalian sirtuins—emerging

roles in physiology, aging, and calorie restriction. Genes Dev. Nov 1 2006;20(21):2913-2921.

277. Baur JA, Sinclair DA. Therapeutic potential of resveratrol: the in vivo evidence. Nat Rev Drug Discov. 2006;5(6):493-506.

278. Dalsky GP. Effect of exercise on bone: permissive influence of estrogen and calcium. Medicine and science in sports and exercise. 1990;22(3):281-285.

279. Gorostiaga EM, Walter CB, Foster C, Hickson RC. Uniqueness of interval and continuous training at the same maintained exercise intensity. European Journal of Applied Physiology and Occupational Physiology. 1991;63(2):101-107.

280. Harmer AR, McKenna MJ, Sutton JR, et al. Skeletal muscle metabolic and ionic adaptations during intense exercise following sprint training in humans. Journal of Applied Physiology. 2000;89(5):1793-1803.

281. Meckel Y, Eliakim A, Seraev M, et al. The Effect of a Brief Sprint Interval Exercise on Growth Factors and Inflammatory Mediators. The Journal of Strength & Conditioning Research. 2009;23(1):225-230 210.1519/JSC.1510b1013e3181876a3181879a.

282. Paton CD, Hopkins WG. Combining explosive and high-resistance training improves performance in competitive cyclists. Journal of strength and conditioning research / National Strength & Conditioning Association. Nov 2005;19(4):826-830.

283. Lunn WR, Finn JA, Axtell RS. Effects of sprint interval training and body weight reduction on power to weight ratio in experienced cyclists. Journal of strength and conditioning research / National Strength & Conditioning Association. Jul 2009;23(4):1217-1224.

284. Hafstad AD, Boardman NT, Lund J, et al. High intensity interval training alters substrate utilization and reduces oxygen consumption in the heart. Journal of Applied Physiology. November 1, 2011 2011;111(5):1235-1241.

285. Sneyd MJ, Cox B. A comparison of trends in melanoma mortality in New Zealand and Australia: the two countries with the highest melanoma incidence and mortality

in the world. BMC Cancer. Aug 6 2013;13(1):372.

286. Rosso S, Sera F, Segnan N, Zanetti R. Sun exposure prior to diagnosis is associated with improved survival in melanoma patients: results from a long-term follow-up study of Italian patients. Eur J Cancer. Jun 2008;44(9):1275-1281.

287. Berwick M, Armstrong BK, Ben-Porat L, et al. Sun Exposure and Mortality From Melanoma. Journal of the National Cancer Institute. February 2, 2005 2005;97(3):195-199.

288. Gandini S, Sera F, Cattaruzza MS, et al. Meta-analysis of risk factors for cutaneous melanoma: II. Sun exposure. Eur J Cancer. 2005;41(1):45-60.

289. Shipman AR, Clark AB, Levell NJ. Sunnier European countries have lower melanoma mortality. Clinical and Experimental Dermatology. 2011;36(5):544-547.

290. Purdue MP, Freeman LE, Anderson WF, Tucker MA. Recent trends in incidence of cutaneous melanoma among US Caucasian young adults. J Invest Dermatol. Dec 2008;128(12):2905-2908.

291. Planta MB. Sunscreen and Melanoma: Is Our Prevention Message Correct? The Journal of the American Board of Family Medicine. November 1, 2011 2011;24(6):735-739.

292. Zanetti R, Franceschi S, Rosso S, Colonna S, Bidoli E. Cutaneous melanoma and sunburns in childhood in a southern European population. Eur J Cancer. 1992;28A(6-7):1172-1176.

293. Dennis LK, Vanbeek MJ, Beane Freeman LE, Smith BJ, Dawson DV, Coughlin JA. Sunburns and risk of cutaneous melanoma: does age matter? A comprehensive meta-analysis. Ann Epidemiol. Aug 2008;18(8):614-627.

294. Bataille V, Winnett A, Sasieni P, Newton Bishop JA, Cuzick J. Exposure to the sun and sunbeds and the risk of cutaneous melanoma in the UK: a case-control study. Eur J Cancer. Feb 2004;40(3):429-435.

295. Wolf P, Quehenberger F, Mullegger R, Stranz B, Kerl H. Phenotypic markers, sunlight-related factors and sunscreen use in patients with cutaneous melanoma: an Austrian case-control study. Melanoma Res. Aug

1998;8(4):370-378.

296. Bastuji-Garin S, Diepgen TL. Cutaneous malignant melanoma, sun exposure, and sunscreen use: epidemiological evidence. British Journal of Dermatology. 2002;146:24-30.

297. S. Lal JB, A.K.Singh, P.K. Shukla. Saree Cancer: The Malignant Changes in Chronic Irritation. Journal of Clinical and Diagnostic Research [serial online]. July 23 2013 2012;6(5):896-898.

298. Surveillance Epidemiology and End Results (SEER). 2013; seer.cancer.gov. Accessed June 1, 2013, 2013.

299. Anderson LN, Cotterchio M, Kirsh VA, Knight JA. Ultraviolet Sunlight Exposure During Adolescence and Adulthood and Breast Cancer Risk: A Population-based Case-Control Study Among Ontario Women. American Journal of Epidemiology. August 1, 2011 2011;174(3):293-304.

300. John EM, Koo J, Schwartz GG. Sun Exposure and Prostate Cancer Risk: Evidence for a Protective Effect of Early-Life Exposure. Cancer Epidemiology Biomarkers & Prevention. June 1, 2007 2007;16(6):1283-1286.

301. Garland CF, Garland FC. Do sunlight and vitamin D reduce the likelihood of colon cancer? International Journal of Epidemiology. April 1, 2006 2006;35(2):217-220.

302. Mohr SB, Garland CF, Gorham ED, Grant WB, Garland FC. Could ultraviolet B irradiance and vitamin D be associated with lower incidence rates of lung cancer? Journal of Epidemiology and Community Health. January 1, 2008 2008;62(1):69-74.

303. Holick MF. Vitamin D: importance in the prevention of cancers, type 1 diabetes, heart disease, and osteoporosis. The American Journal of Clinical Nutrition. March 1, 2004 2004;79(3):362-371.

304. Holick MF, Biancuzzo RM, Chen TC, et al. Vitamin D2 is as effective as vitamin D3 in maintaining circulating concentrations of 25-hydroxyvitamin D. The Journal of clinical endocrinology and metabolism. Mar 2008;93(3):677-681.

305. Holick MF, MacLaughlin JA, Doppelt SH. Regulation

of cutaneous previtamin D3 photosynthesis in man: skin pigment is not an essential regulator. Science. Feb 6 1981;211(4482):590-593.

306. Pittaway JK, Ahuja KDK, Beckett JM, Bird M-L, Robertson IK, Ball MJ. Make Vitamin D While the Sun Shines, Take Supplements When It Doesn't: A Longitudinal, Observational Study of Older Adults in Tasmania, Australia. PLoS ONE. 2013;8(3):e59063.

307. Taha SA, Dost SM, Sedrani SH. 25-Hydroxyvitamin D and total calcium: extraordinarily low plasma concentrations in Saudi mothers and their neonates. Pediatr Res. Aug 1984;18(8):739-741.

308. Fischer TW, Sweatman TW, Semak I, Sayre RM, Wortsman J, Slominski A. Constitutive and UV-induced metabolism of melatonin in keratinocytes and cell-free systems. The FASEB Journal. July 1, 2006 2006;20(9):1564-1566.

309. Reiter RJ, Melchiorri D, Sewerynek E, et al. A review of the evidence supporting melatonin's role as an antioxidant. Journal of Pineal Research. 1995;18(1):1-11.

310. Molis TM, Spriggs LL, Hill SM. Modulation of estrogen receptor mRNA expression by melatonin in MCF-7 human breast cancer cells. Molecular Endocrinology. December 1, 1994 1994;8(12):1681-1690.

311. Blask DE. Melatonin, sleep disturbance and cancer risk. Sleep medicine reviews. 2009;13(4):257-264.

312. Giovannucci E, Liu Y, Rimm EB, et al. Prospective Study of Predictors of Vitamin D Status and Cancer Incidence and Mortality in Men. Journal of the National Cancer Institute. 5 April 2006 2006;98(7):451-459.

313. Lappe JM, Travers-Gustafson D, Davies KM, Recker RR, Heaney RP. Vitamin D and calcium supplementation reduces cancer risk: results of a randomized trial. The American journal of clinical nutrition. Jun 2007;85(6):1586-1591.

314. Skowronski RJ, Peehl DM, Feldman D. Vitamin D and prostate cancer: 1,25 dihydroxyvitamin D3 receptors and actions in human prostate cancer cell lines. Endocrinology. May 1993;132(5):1952-1960.

315. Garland C, Barrett-Connor E, Rossof A, Shekelle R,

Criqui M, Paul O. Dietary Vitamin D and Calcium and Risk of Colorectal Cancer: A 19-year Prospective Stufy in Men. The Lancet. 1985;325(8424):307-309.

316. Ma Y, Zhang P, Wang F, Yang J, Liu Z, Qin H. Association between vitamin D and risk of colorectal cancer: a systematic review of prospective studies. Journal of clinical oncology : official journal of the American Society of Clinical Oncology. Oct 1 2011;29(28):3775-3782.

317. Ford ES, Zhao G, Tsai J, Li C. Vitamin D and all-cause mortality among adults in USA: findings from the National Health and Nutrition Examination Survey Linked Mortality Study. International Journal of Epidemiology. August 1, 2011 2011;40(4):998-1005.

318. Yamshchikov AV, Desai NS, Blumberg HM, Ziegler TR, Tangpricha V. Vitamin D for treatment and prevention of infectious diseases: a systematic review of randomized controlled trials. Endocrine practice : official journal of the American College of Endocrinology and the American Association of Clinical Endocrinologists. Jul-Aug 2009;15(5):438-449.

319. Grant WB. Solar ultraviolet irradiance and cancer incidence and mortality. Adv Exp Med Biol. 2008;624:16-30.

320. Schöttker B, Haug U, Schomburg L, et al. Strong associations of 25-hydroxyvitamin D concentrations with all-cause, cardiovascular, cancer, and respiratory disease mortality in a large cohort study. The American Journal of Clinical Nutrition. April 1, 2013 2013.

321. van der Rhee H, Coebergh JW, de Vries E. Is prevention of cancer by sun exposure more than just the effect of vitamin D? A systematic review of epidemiological studies. European journal of cancer (Oxford, England : 1990). 2013;49(6):1422-1436.

322. Nickel A, Wohlrab W. Melatonin protects human keratinocytes from UVB irradiation by light absorption. Arch Dermatol Res. Jul 2000;292(7):366-368.

323. Bowell RJ, Warren A, Redmond I. Formation of cave salts and utilization by elephants in the Mount Elgon region, Kenya. Geological Society, London, Special Publications. January 1, 1996 1996;113(1):63-79.

324. Chobanian AV, Bakris GL, Black HR, et al. Seventh Report of the Joint National Committee on Prevention, Detection, Evaluation, and Treatment of High Blood Pressure. Hypertension. December 1, 2003 2003;42(6):1206-1252.

325. Heaney RP. Role of Dietary Sodium in Osteoporosis. Journal of the American College of Nutrition. June 2006 2006;25(suppl 3):271S-276S.

326. He FJ, MacGregor GA. Effect of longer-term modest salt reduction on blood pressure. Cochrane database of systematic reviews. 2004(3):CD004937.

327. Cook NR, Cutler JA, Obarzanek E, et al. Long term effects of dietary sodium reduction on cardiovascular disease outcomes: observational follow-up of the trials of hypertension prevention (TOHP). BMJ. 2007-04-26 00:00:00 2007;334(7599):885.

328. Jurgens G, Graudal NA. Effects of low sodium diet versus high sodium diet on blood pressure, renin, aldosterone, catecholamines, cholesterols, and triglyceride. Cochrane database of systematic reviews. 2004(1):CD004022.

329. Stolarz-Skrzypek K KTTL, et al. FAtal and nonfatal outcomes, incidence of hypertension, and blood pressure changes in relation to urinary sodium excretion. JAMA: The Journal of the American Medical Association. 2011;305(17):1777-1785.

330. Alderman MH, Cohen H, Madhavan S. Dietary sodium intake and mortality: the National Health and Nutrition Examination Survey (NHANES I). Lancet. Mar 14 1998;351(9105):781-785.

331. Cohen HW, Hailpern SM, Fang J, Alderman MH. Sodium intake and mortality in the NHANES II follow-up study. The American journal of medicine. Mar 2006;119(3):275 e277-214.

332. Cohen HW, Hailpern SM, Alderman MH. Sodium intake and mortality follow-up in the Third National Health and Nutrition Examination Survey (NHANES III). Journal of general internal medicine. Sep 2008;23(9):1297-1302.

333. Paterna S, Gaspare P, Fasullo S, Sarullo FM, Di Pasquale

P. Normal-sodium diet compared with low-sodium diet in compensated congestive heart failure: is sodium an old enemy or a new friend? Clin Sci (Lond). Feb 2008;114(3):221-230.

334. Ekinci EI, Clarke S, Thomas MC, et al. Dietary Salt Intake and Mortality in Patients With Type 2 Diabetes. Diabetes Care. March 1, 2011 2011;34(3):703-709.

335. Graudal Na GAMGP. Effects of sodium restriction on blood pressure, renin, aldosterone, catecholamines, cholesterols, and triglyceride: A meta-analysis. JAMA: The Journal of the American Medical Association. 1998;279(17):1383-1391.

336. Folkow B. Critical review of studies on salt and hypertension. Clinical and experimental hypertension. Part A, Theory and practice. 1992;14(1-2):1-14.

337. Sharp RL. Role of Sodium in Fluid Homeostasis with Exercise. Journal of the American College of Nutrition. June 2006 2006;25(suppl 3):231S-239S.

338. Skøtt P, Hother-Nielsen O, Bruun N, et al. Effects of insulin on kidney function and sodium excretion in healthy subjects. Diabetologia. 1989;32(9):694-699.

339. DeFronzo RA. The effect of insulin on renal sodium metabolism. A review with clinical implications. Diabetologia. Sep 1981;21(3):165-171.

340. Garg R, Williams GH, Hurwitz S, Brown NJ, Hopkins PN, Adler GK. Low-salt diet increases insulin resistance in healthy subjects. Metabolism. 2011;60(7):965-968.

341. Prada PO, Coelho MS, Zecchin HG, et al. Low salt intake modulates insulin signaling, JNK activity and IRS-1ser307 phosphorylation in rat tissues. Journal of Endocrinology. June 1, 2005 2005;185(3):429-437.

342. Feldman RD, Schmidt ND. Moderate dietary salt restriction increases vascular and systemic insulin resistance. American journal of hypertension. Jun 1999;12(6):643-647.

343. Alderman MH. Salt, Blood Pressure, and Human Health. Hypertension. November 1, 2000 2000;36(5):890-893.

344. Westman EC, Yancy WS, Jr., Mavropoulos JC, Marquart M, McDuffie JR. The effect of a low-carbohydrate, keto-

genic diet versus a low-glycemic index diet on glycemic control in type 2 diabetes mellitus. Nutr Metab (Lond). 2008;5:36.

345. Noakes TD. The hyponatremia of exercise. International journal of sport nutrition. Sep 1992;2(3):205-228.

346. Mtabaji JP, Nara Y, Moriguchi Y, Yamori Y. Diet and Hypertension in Tanzania. Journal of Cardiovascular Pharmacology. 1990;16:S3-S5.

347. Americans Consume Too Much Sodium (Salt) http://www.cdc.gov/features/dssodium/. 2011; http://www.cdc.gov/features/dssodium/.

348. Logan AG. Dietary Sodium Intake and Its Relation to Human Health: A Summary of the Evidence. Journal of the American College of Nutrition. June 2006 2006;25(3):165-169.

349. Sodium Intake in Populations: Assessment of Evidence: The National Academies Press; 2013.

350. Geleijnse JM, Witteman JCM, Bak AAA, Breijen JHd, Grobbee DE. Reduction in blood pressure with a low sodium, high potassium, high magnesium salt in older subjects with mild to moderate hypertension. BMJ. 1994-08-13 00:00:00 1994;309(6952):436-440.

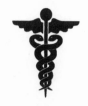

ABOUT THE AUTHOR

COLIN CHAMP

Dr. Champ is a board-certified practicing radiation oncologist and assistant professor at the University of Pittsburgh Cancer Institute and University of Pittsburgh Medical Center. He researches cancer treatment as well as diet and nutrition extensively and has been invited to lecture on the topic around the country and world. He is one of the few physicians invited to present academic Oncology Grand Rounds as a resident, an honor usually reserved for experts after years or decades in the field.

As only a resident, he published over 20 peer-reviewed articles, started a health and fitness website and company, and co-hosted a podcast that was top-ranked in the U.S., England, and Australia. He has been featured in the Boston Globe, The Gupta Guide with Sanjay Gupta, the National Cancer Institute at the National Institute of Health, and the American Society of Clinical Oncology newsletter, to name only a few.